HAVE YOUR CAKE

AND

LOSE WEIGHT TOO!

DANELLE WOLFORD

www.weedemandreap.com

Published by Archangel Ink
Copyright © 2013 Weed 'em & Reap, LLC
www.weedemandreap.com
ISBN 1499709625
ISBN-13 978-1499709629

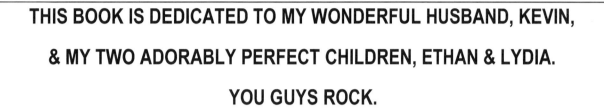

THIS BOOK IS DEDICATED TO MY WONDERFUL HUSBAND, KEVIN,

& MY TWO ADORABLY PERFECT CHILDREN, ETHAN & LYDIA.

YOU GUYS ROCK.

DISCLAIMER AND COPYRIGHT INFORMATION

ABOUT THE AUTHOR

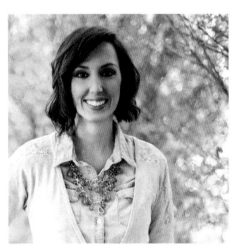

It was two months after her second back surgery, and things still hadn't improved for DaNelle Wolford. At only 29 years old and her whole life ahead of her, she knew that something had to be done. It was then that DaNelle decided to try something radically different from the harsh diets and attempts to deny herself of foods that she craved. She turned to what others were calling "real food." After years of controlling her portions and trying to force down barely edible rabbit food with less than mediocre results, DaNelle embraced real food and found the secret to weight loss & healing. Not only did she find that she could eat dessert every day, she also found that life was enjoyable once again! As if her body was yearning for this lifestyle all along, she was able to lose all of her excess fat and heal without taking diet pills, counting calories, avoiding yummy foods, or doing any unwanted exercise. DaNelle's down to earth personality and charming dialogue will encourage you to finally find the life you want by eating real food that is both nourishing and satisfying. Whether you're hoping to lose weight or heal your body from problems your doctors don't seem to have an answer for, you will love DaNelle's simple method to finally losing the weight and finding freedom from those crappy restrictive diets.

TABLE OF CONTENTS

Introduction: A Delicious Way to Lose Weight

What if I said you could lose weight eating fried chicken, mashed potatoes with gravy, and a side of butter green beans? Would you believe me is I saud you could look forward to delicious pizza & soda on the weekends? Could you imagine what it would feel like to eat dessert every night guilt-free?

Most people think these types of food are not synonymous with weight loss. Why is that, do you think? And why, for heaven sakes, haven't we won the war on weight loss? I believe the problem lies in fad diets. With every new diet comes more confusion. We now believe that the **only way** to lose weight is to jump on one of the common diet plans. We jump on either the low-carb, low-fat, or low-protein train. We watch documentaries, read diet books, listen to diet gurus, and come to the conclusion that our only salvation is through eating rabbit food all day, every day. Well, take a seat people, because I'm here to tell you that ALL you have learned about losing weight and maintaining that weight loss is WRONG! Are you shocked? I'd be surprised if you weren't. The problem with all those diets, all that nonsense, is that despite all that ridiculous food restriction, everybody just seems to be getting fatter.

I'm not a nutritionist, nor a practitioner. While I do have a background in nursing, I don't carry any special title behind my name. But through 10 years of personal experience and research on the matter, I believe I have discovered the TRUE SOLUTION to WEIGHT LOSS. And you may be surprised to find out it's much, much simpler and more satisfying than you think.

I Successfully Lost 35 Pounds

How did I do it? Well, let's first go over what I DID NOT DO:

- I DID NOT take weight-loss pills.
- I DID NOT exercise excessively.
- I DID NOT count one single calorie or use portion control.
- I DID NOT eat low-fat, low-carb, or low-protein.

Well, then what did I do?

I ate REAL FOOD, WHOLE & UNPROCESSED. I also...

- ATE whenever the heck I wanted to, even late at night.
- ATE dessert every. single. day.
- ATE foods I desired, just substituted bad ingredients for good.
- ATE all food groups, in a balance my body naturally desired.

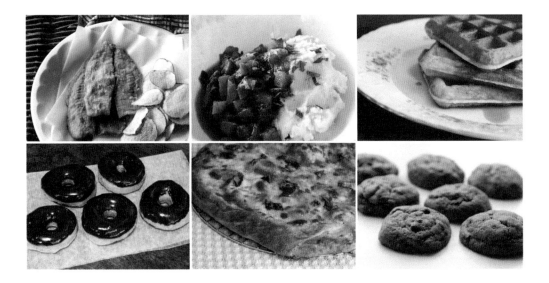

And because you're pretty much the coolest person ever for reading this book, I'm gonna show you how to do it, too!

Trust me, I know how it feels to be in "that place." Never fitting in your clothes, never wanting to buy new fat clothes, never understanding why the weight won't come off. Always losing weight with a diet fad, only to gain it all back again, plus some. My hope is that you'll receive some inspiration from my words and find that balance your body has been longing for. Well, either that or you'll at least fit into those skinny jeans of yours. Life is about learning. Learn some stuff, do it, and reap the results!

Chapter 1: Real Food -- How it all got messed up.

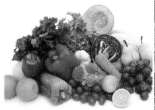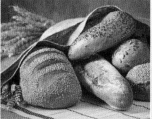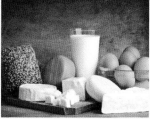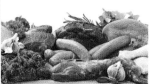

What comes to your mind when I say the phrase "real food?" I htink of things like whole milk, butter, cream, farm fresh eggsm warm bread, fresh garden vegetables, whole cuts of meat like steak, lamb chops or bacon, and hearty soups made with real homemade broth. If you thought of those same foods too, then you are right! Traditional food has nourished people literally for thousands of years, and is something your ancestors would recognize. Ironically, a typical grocery store carries only 10% real food and most is found in the produce department. The rest is highly processed and shouldn't even be considered "food." I am amazed at what is called "food" in our grocery stores today. Yogurt in a tube, cookies in a tub, protein in a powder, & 100 calorie packs of whatever – what would your great-grandma think?

If I interviewed 10 random people and asked them to name a healthy food, they'd probably all say the same thing – vegetables. In their minds, plants are what we are always told to eat more of. "Eat more fruits and vegetables," says our doctor. "Be sure to get your 5-a-day!" says every nutrition poster we encounter from kindergarten on up. Naturally, we jump to the conclusion that before our ancestors started butchering animals, there must have been societies that meditated all say, survived merely on fruits, vegetables, and grains, and therefore lived in perfectly harmonious communities. "Fruits and vegetables are the key to everything!" we say to ourselves, as we choke down another celery stick.

This idea -- this illusion -- that we stem from plant-eating great-great-great-great grandparents is WRONG. Our history, our way of life before the industrialization of food, was centered on ALL foods – **vegetables, fruits, meat, dairy, and grains.** Today because of diet myths, incomplete scientific studies, and conspiring corporations funding those studies, we are lost in the abyss of health dogma. It seems like everything is bad for us, then it's miraculously touted for its health benefits only to be placed back on the black list again a couple years later. How can we find true answers in a time of so much confusion? The answer?

We must look back at the wisdom of our ancestors.

In the 1930s, a Cleveland dentist named Dr. Weston A. Price sought to research traditional diets in an effort to gain understanding as to why so many Americans were suffering physical degeneration. A devout Christian, Price married Florence Anthony and founded his dental practice in the town of Grand Forks, North Dakota. Unfortunately, his life didn't turn out as he had planned. Weston Price contracted Typhoid fever and nearly died. In his emaciated condition, a dear friend of Dr. Price's and a man of great wisdom, William Delmage, took Price away from his home and provided a retreat at Lake Mazinaw. This friend camped and fished with Price, and fed him a diet of salmon, trout, huckleberries, wild raspberries, and small game along with a good dose of fresh air, sunshine and good water. Weston described this retreat as "a place God had chosen to teach man a lesson in humility." He vowed to return one day and build a large cabin so that other people might share such an experience as he did. Later in his life, he fulfilled that vow. Dr. Price learned early on in his life that he didn't have anything if he didn't have his health.

Dr. Weston A. Price later founded the research department of the National Dental Association, which later became the American Dental Association. **When Weston and Florence Price's only child died of an infected root canal, his interest into the cause of tooth decay was intensified.** He noticed that the children in his office suffered from cavities, tooth decay, and crooked teeth, while the parents of these children had good oral health. How could this be? What was causing this sudden rise in poor oral health and degenerative disease that his own child had died of?

After spending years in the laboratory studying clinical theories, Dr. Weston Price found that instead of looking for **"injurious factors" causing bad health**, he needed to find **"essential factors" that were missing** from the Standard American Diet in the 1930s. Basically, he needed a control group. He needed to find people that were immune to physical degeneration and find out what they were doing RIGHT.

Price spent the next 9 years of his life traveling around the world with his wife, Florence, and a team of scientists. His studies of traditional cultures included:

- The Swiss of Switzerland
- The Gaelics in the Outer and Inner Hebrides
- The Eskimos of Alaska
- The Indians in the far North, West, and Central Canada, Western United States & Florida
- The Melanesians and Polynesians on eight archipelagos of the Southern Pacific
- The tribes in eastern and central Africa
- The Aborigines of Australia

- The Malay tribes on the islands north of Australia
- The Maori of New Zealand
- The cultures of Peru

Without bias and without financial support from friends or colleagues, Price (along with his wife) spent 9 years searching the globe...

"Rejecting all proffered aid and commercial pressure, his independent and unbiased research was entirely financed by the income of his own practice. He steadfastly held to a conviction that it was the only way to follow the trail to the true facts with integrity."

-Donald Delmage Fawcett, a grand-nephew of Dr. Weston A. Price

Dr. Price's trail of research led him to so-called "primitive races" that had thrived on the same soil for thousands of years. Why had Americans suffered declining health in merely a few decades? His extensive studies revealed that **traditional cultures experienced a high immunity to many degenerative diseases as long as they were isolated from modern civilization and subsequent modern diets.** Also, they were more than just healthy; they were gorgeous, had zero cavities, broad jaws and straight teeth, strong backs, amazing fertility, longevity, and VITALITY! When an individual from one of these cultures left their traditional diet and ate modern processed foods, however, poor health would usually present itself in the next generation.

It became clear that including modern, processed foods in our diet was extremely detrimental to our health.

Since the early 1900s, our food has rapidly changed from flourishing in home gardens, to growing in a farmer's field, to being created in a lab. We are offered machine processed, DNA spliced, hazmat suit handled frankenfood. And somehow, everybody seems cool with it. Until now. More and more people are wising up and realizing the benefits of doing it "the old fashioned way." They are also realizing it tastes a heck of a lot better. And BONUS, their weight loss & health issues are resolved. Real food sees air, sunshine, and soil. Real food is fresh, alive, and full of nutrients your body needs. Real food is not even really a diet, it's a way of living! And let me tell you, it's a delicious & satisfying place to be!

When the industrialization of food changed EVERYTHING:

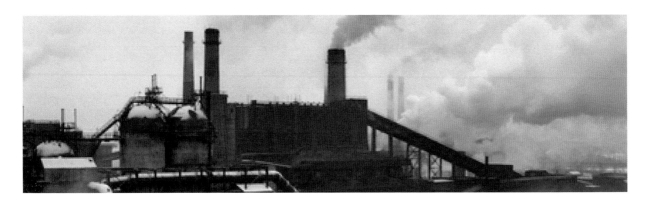

In the late 1800s, the company Procter & Gamble were doin' mighty fine growing & harvesting cotton. The cottonseed, a bothersome byproduct of cotton, became so numerous that Procter & Gamble decided to see if there was anything –*anything*- they could make from the cottonseed to increase their profit. It seemed awfully wasteful to throw pounds and pounds of that cottonseed away.

They found after intense processing -- which included heating & pressing that pesky cotton seed – that they were able to extract oil. And it cost Procter & Gamble next to NOTHING to produce it. An easily rancid and unstable fat, cottonseed oil was rendered stable and long lasting by adding the process of hydrogenation. When the cottonseed oil cooled, it looked exactly like lard.

They called it **Crisco.**

Now, this is a crucial point in our history, folks. Procter & Gamble's decision to market and sell cottonseed oil (Crisco) has perhaps caused more physical sickness & suffering than we could probably ever quantify. Procter & Gamble sneakily marketed Crisco as a cheaper and "healthier" fat. Lard was touted as unhealthy or smelly. Procter & Gamble even gave away free cookbooks with every purchase of Crisco. Now wasn't that nice of them? The cookbooks were full of common recipes, but instead of lard or butter, Crisco was listed as the cooking fat. It's incredibly sad really, how successful they were at convincing people to turn away from the traditional use of lard, butter, and tallow. Even sadder, you probably eat cottonseed oil every single day. Why? **Cottonseed oil is in almost EVERY PACKAGED or PROCESSED food** in your store. Chips, cereals, cookies, granola bars, tortillas, crackers, breads, salad dressings, mayonnaise, pasta sauces, fast food, soaps, shampoos, conditioners, makeup, lipstick, **EVERYTHING.**

Why is cottonseed oil used in almost every product? Because it's CHEAP to produce and it saves big food corporations lots of MONEY!

According to the book, The Happiness Diet:

"Never before had Procter & Gamble -- or any company for that matter -- put so much marketing support or advertising dollars behind a product. They hired the J. Walter Thompson Agency, America's first full service advertising agency staffed by real artists and professional writers. Samples of Crisco were mailed to grocers, restaurants, nutritionists, and home economists. Eight alternative marketing strategies were tested in different cities and their impacts calculated and compared. Doughnuts were fried in Crisco and handed out in the streets. Women who purchased the new industrial fat got a free cookbook of Crisco recipes. It opened with the line, 'The culinary world is revising its entire cookbook on account of the advent of Crisco, a new and altogether different cooking fat.' Recipes for asparagus soup, baked salmon with Colbert sauce, stuffed beets, curried cauliflower, and tomato sandwiches all called for three to four tablespoons of Crisco."

And why is Crisco/cottonseed oil so bad for us, you ask?

Well, for starters, cotton is not considered a food crop by the FDA, and therefore is NOT regulated on the amount of pesticides that can be sprayed. In fact, more pesticides are sprayed on cotton **THAN ANY OTHER CROP.**

The Happiness Diet *adds*:

"Before processing, cottonseed oil is cloudy red and bitter to the taste because of a natural phytochemical called gossypol... and is toxic to most animals, causing dangerous spikes in the body's potassium levels, organ damage, and paralysis. An issue of Popular Science from the era sums up the evolution of cottonseed nicely: "What was garbage in 1860 was fertilizer in 1870, cattle feed in 1880, and table food and many things else in 1890."

Did you know that cottonseed oil has over 50% poly-unsaturated fatty acids?! Also known as polyunsaturated fat, Omega-6 fatty acids produce a high inflammatory response in our bodies. Although we do need a teensy-tiny amount of Omega-6 fatty acids for health, too much of it promotes disease & sickness. The other thing to note here is that the fat found in cottonseed oil (Omega-6 fatty acids), could not be produced in your kitchen. A modern, processed oil, indeed.

Sadly, with the industrialization of food came disease. Before the industrialization of food, before Procter & Gamble came up with their elusive scheme, heart disease was nearly unheard of. It was rare. Obsolete. Soon after the infiltration of Crisco/cottonseed oil into our food supply came the rise of inflammation & a variety of diseases -- Heart Disease, Diabetes, Infertility, Multiple Sclerosis, Cancer & Autism to name a few. Now these diseases are so common, they're household names.

A common argument arises…"Maybe our ancestors suffered from these ailments but didn't have the medical technology to diagnose them. Maybe they were fat and sick too."

Luckily for us, we have traditional cultures who eat a traditional diet TODAY and are FREE from disease, proving to us that there IS a formula to avoiding disease & obesity.

> *"Aboriginal populations, who do not consume foods that humans are not adapted for, have a disease panorama that is quite different from people in the Western world. Yet, this is not due to a lack of older persons. Myocardial infarctions, sudden cardiac death from stroke and heart failure are uncommon or missing altogether in aboriginal peoples. The risk factor levels are also very beneficial. Blood pressure is low and does not increase with age as it does for us. Being overweight is not common, and everyone is very thin. Type 2 diabetes and insulin resistance do not seem to be present either. When traditional ethnic groups switch to a Western lifestyle, they suffer from exactly the same ills as we do, including abdominal obesity, hypertension, diabetes, and cardiovascular disease. The spread of stroke after urbanization in Africa and Papua New Guinea is only one of several noticeable examples."*
>
> *-Lindeberg, Staffan*, <u>Food and Western Disease</u>

In many studies performed on traditional cultures, the answer is clear. Traditional, real food will keep us free from disease & obesity. One by one, when each family strayed from real food and towards conveniently packaged modern food, with it came disease & obesity. We need only to turn back the dial a bit, remember our roots, and rediscover our natural diet.

Chapter 2: Traditional Wisdom vs. Modern Interpretations

One of the most common questions when talking about the wisdom of traditional diets is, *"Didn't people way back then drop dead at 40? They were barbaric, ate a lot of meat & fat, and had a shorter life expectancy, right?"*

WRONG! **Life expectancy is not a recorded number of the age people died**, but rather an average of all deaths. High infant mortality rates before 1900 skewed the numbers. The high infant mortality rate before the 1900s was due to unclean conditions and poor medical care. Subsequently, life expectancy numbers before the year 1900 gets easily knocked down to a low life number. Because infant mortality rates decreased as medical technology increased, the average life expectancy for men in 1907 was 45.6 years, in 1957 it was 66.4, and in 2007 it reached 75.5. The increase of life expectancy is due to a decreasing infant mortality rate, which was 9.99% in 1907, 2.63% in 1957, and 0.68% in 2007.

The truth is the human lifespan has been consistent for more than 2,000 years!

"The inclusion of infant mortality rates in calculating life expectancy creates the mistaken impression that earlier generations died at a young age; Americans were not dying en masse at the age of 46 in 1907. The fact is that the maximum human lifespan — a concept often confused with "life expectancy" — has remained more or less the same for thousands of years. The idea that our ancestors routinely died young (say, at age 40) has no basis in scientific fact. When Socrates died at the age of 70 around 399 B.C., he did not die of old age but instead by execution. It is ironic that ancient Greeks lived into their 70s and older, while more than 2,000 years later modern Americans aren't living much longer."

- Benjamin Radford, <u>Bad Science Column</u>

Just for curiosity, I decided to research **my own ancestral line** as well as **my husband's ancestral line** to find out how long our very own ancestors lived…

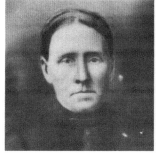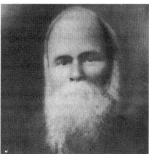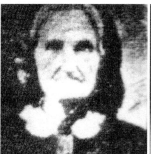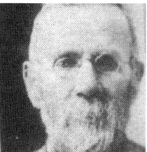

• My husband's great-great-great-great grandfather Augustas Oliver Artemas Stowell, was born June 4th, 1783 and died August 23, 1860 at **age 77.**

- My husband's great-great-great-great grandmother Mary Stephens Holmes, was born Sept. 15th, 1797 and died Nov. 20th, 1885 at **age 88.**
- My great-great-great-great grandfather James Monroe Lindsey, was born December 30th, 1829 and died January 9, 1912 at **age 83.**
- My great-great-great-great grandmother Mary Sarah Ann Little, was born July 2nd, 1832 and died March 5th, 1910 at **age 78.**

An excerpt from **my great-great-great grandmother Martha Lindsey's journal** shows the amazing VITALITY the traditional diet brings…

"The day & night before school started in 1901, I worked one hundred buttonholes and sewed on one hundred buttons, trying to finish up the children's school clothes. I was still sewing at dawn. I milked the cows and fixed breakfast. I worked all morning about the house and cooked dinner. Then that afternoon I gave birth to my **tenth child.**"

Learning from the past to thrive in the future…

I'm not trying to offend any scientists out there, but let's just admit that nutritional science is pretty much still in its infantile stage. The effect diet plays on the body is a relatively new arena, with the earliest studies just starting in the 20th century. Since that time, there have been countless "official statements" from top scientists on what particular food is beneficial only to be touted as unhealthy in the next study. The same scientists that used to tell us coconut oil was bad are now telling us it is good. One year we are told that it's the egg whites that are bad, but the next year it's the yolks that are the culprits. Today, the American Heart Association tells us to eat margarine and avoid butter. Seriously?! Eat highly processed inflammatory trans-fats and avoid nourishing, vitamin-rich butter?!

The modern interpretation of a healthy diet is confusing and misleading. What's more, scientists often study single nutrients or vitamins without recognizing the importance of whole foods. And while I'm not a huge conspiracy theorist, I have to say it's still very fishy once you find out who is funding these "studies."

The wisdom from our ancestors is priceless.

Our ancestors didn't worry about heart disease, cancer, or diabetes. They didn't fear Alzheimer's or Parkinson's disease. These diseases were so incredibly rare before the 1900s that they didn't need scientists to solve any mystery. There was no mystery! Our ancestors simply ate food – real food - and were nourished. Sure, there was illness and life was not perfect. But chronic degenerative diseases were unheard of.

The leading cause of death before 1900 was one of four things: infancy death, death from childbirth, death from infections, & death from accidents. Today, the leading causes of death are heart disease & cancer. Clearly, there's something we need to change.

Following a traditional diet will give us optimal health. Seasonal fruits & vegetables, grains, milk, butter, cream, meat, seafood, eggs – all in the best form possible – is the key to weight loss and disease reversal.

Avoiding fake foods, like store bought crackers, cookies, cereals, granola bars, and protein mixes -- as much as possible (without stressing about it too much) – is the key to keeping our bodies clean & toxin-free.

Born n' raised in the LOW-FAT ERA

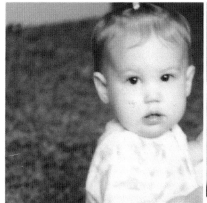 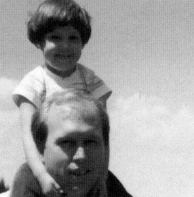 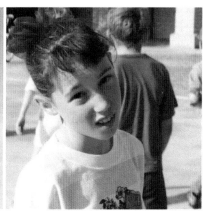

I was born to a family of all girls, and as such, took my role as the self-appointed tomboy very seriously. I spent my days playing outside and was an absolute expert in tree-climbing – especially when I was in trouble. I grew up during a time when children actually loved to play outside. Remember when your curfew was determined by the glow of porch lights? Those were the days! Although I was raised to work hard & play hard, I was also raised in the 80's, a time when low-fat was the thing to do! My mother made homemade bread and refused to buy sugar cereal, but we drank skim milk and avoided high-fat foods like everybody else in America at the time. Because a low-fat diet deprived us of essential nutrients, we often broke our "healthy" rules and ate Oreos, mac n' cheese out of a box, & Pringles.

My story probably sounds a lot like yours. I didn't think much about healthy eating (or my weight for that matter) until I was fat & sick. Do you remember thinking you were overweight in high school and then when you look back at those pictures, you wish you could look like that **now**?

Well, that was me, too.

I am 5'6", and when I married my husband, I was 128 lbs. It seemed like only months after we were married, I gained 25+ lbs. and all of the sudden I was 155. Size 12-14 jeans! I blame it on the husband. Just kidding. Actually, I should blame it on hospital food during nursing school (because it was free YOU GUYS) - boxed brownies and frozen food. Lots of frozen food. Because it was cheap, and we were poor. I had no clue what it meant to truly be healthy.

I assumed eating healthy meant I needed to eat salad all day or at least go back to my childhood of low-fatness.

My quest for health began once my health started to decline. After nursing school and the birth of my two children, I had horrible back pain, resulting in many chiropractic & physical therapy visits, which did nothing to ease my pain. Convinced I had no control over my health, I resorted to back surgery, and after that didn't work, I resorted to….yes, another back surgery. I also began to experience vertigo, a crippling dizziness that left me in bed for days. I was only 24 years old, living a life of pain and disability, with no hope for a better life in the future. Doctors labeled me "too complicated" and after countless specialists and misdiagnoses, I felt like I had no help from the medical world at all. I avoided leaving the house. I spent $10,000 – $15,000 per year on doctors, chiropractors, physical therapists, & alternative medicine specialists. Nothing was working. My lowest point came when at 28 years of age, I bought a wheelchair and applied for a handicapped sign for my car. Another pregnancy was completely out of the question and although we wanted to adopt, I feared being able to even do that. I decided I wasn't going to give up. There had to be *something* I could do to feel better.

In the beginning, I didn't care about my weight - I just wanted to somehow reduce my pain and heal my chronic issues. I started sampling various healthy recipes, but never really committed to a diet that would promote true wellness in my body. I studied REAL FOOD and I knew that it would help with my inflammation and healing. But I was already tired and sick, and it seemed too overwhelming to start a whole lifestyle change. When I decided that doctors weren't going to help me and I stepped into the world of natural healing, I was not prepared for the "internet education" I'd get…

Meat is bad, definitely bad. So acidic and it rots. Did you know you are eating rotting flesh?

Animal fats are bad. They cause heart disease and cancer and diabetes. Plus it'll make you really fat.

Grains are bird food. Humans shouldn't even eat it. Ever. It destroys your gut by the way.

Are you drinking a green smoothie every morning? Well, it's not enough! You need to eat veggies all day if you're even gonna think about getting healthy.

I can't believe you are drinking milk from an animal. That is disgusting! Did you know that humans are the only species that drinks the milk of another species?

To say I was confused is a gross understatement! Two years ago I decided to start with something drastic, something everybody else seemed to be doing…a juice cleanse. I committed to a 30 day cleanse – you heard me right – 30 days! At that point, I was living on pain medication and was experiencing more "bad" days than "good." In fact, I don't think I could even remember what a "good" day felt like.

Looking back, I can't totally slam juice cleanses because I did experience a significant detox in my body. I lost only 8 lbs., but I was also able to detox from pain medication & junk food. I don't usually recommend this for other people and here's why: I don't think the minimal nutrients in fruit & vegetable juices necessarily helped my body as much as the **avoidance of all processed foods during that 30 day juice cleanse.** As my body detoxed from chemicals primarily found in junk food, I was able to become "cleaner," and for that I am thankful. But juice cleansing is a drastic measure, something that can put a lot of stress on your kidneys, liver, thyroid & hormone function, and ultimately, your metabolism. My body definitely suffered during that juice cleansing and that's why I wouldn't recommend it. I had extreme flu-like symptoms, experienced kidney pain, and felt weak & dizzy for most of it. I did cleanse my body, but at a price.

Now I understand that I would have experienced a suitable cleanse just from eating homemade foods and avoiding anything processed, packaged, or chemical-laden. The benefit **of not** doing an extreme juice cleanse is that you can avoid some horrible symptoms and undue stress on your body.

If you are set on still doing a juice cleanse, I would recommend a short one, from 3 days to a week **at the most**. I would also recommend doing a cleanse (whether it be with a juice cleanse or just eating fruits & vegetables) **only during the summer months.** During the summer, high amounts of cooling foods (fruits & vegetables) won't be a stress on your body. But, if you attempt a cleanse during the cold months, a time when your body is craving comfort foods (meat & potatoes) to keep you warm, your body will interpret the cleanse as a stressful experience and you'll gain more weight in the end. When the weather is hot outside, we tend to crave cleansing foods anyway (watermelon, cantaloupe, salads), and your body will naturally do better with a cleanse during these months than it would during cold months. Your metabolism is a fragile thing, one that can be easily thrown off balance by fad diets that are restrictive in nature. Use wisdom before you start any extreme diet.

By the time I was finished with my 30 day juice cleanse, I transitioned to a vegetarian, plant-based diet. I honestly didn't know what else to do and so I relied on fruit, vegetables, nuts, and grains to feed my body. I was losing weight slowly yet steadily on this diet (about 1 lb. a week), but I noticed the weight came back fast if I strayed from this strict diet. I also was definitely NOT feeling better health-wise. I was still experiencing significant inflammation, muscle weakness, fatigue, and depression. I continued on my plant-based path and with each step I became more and more restricted with my diet. After a year on a plant-based diet, not feeling much better than before and with still some weight to lose, I decided to do something even more "drastic."

I decided to turn away from plant-based eating, and just eat REAL FOOD! Within two weeks of bringing back real butter, cream, meat, and desserts, I began to feel amazing! My energy improved, I was happy again, and my health issues started to resolve.

And the most surprising thing of all?

I lost even MORE WEIGHT! From eating BUTTER!

Here I was, eating REAL FOOD, eating from **all food groups** without any major restrictions, and was feeling great! Here's where my research became fun. I started to research *why I was feeling better.* Why had all these foods that were touted as unhealthy, disease-causing, and weight-inducing produced the opposite effect on me? In my research, I found out the most important clue…

TRADITIONAL & sustainable FOODS HEAL – MODERN & unnatural FOODS KILL

But weren't you already eating traditional foods when you were eating plant-based?

-No, actually I wasn't eating a traditional diet when I was eating plant-based. I was eating a restrictive, modern interpretation of a healthy diet, but the diet that societies have thrived on for centuries? IT DEFINITELY WASN'T PLANT-BASED. What have traditional societies successfully thrived on for thousands of years? The answer is ALL FOODS including meat (yes even red meat, bacon, and lamb chops), dairy (cream, butter, whole milk, and yogurt), seafood, grains, fruits, and vegetables.

REAL FOOD CHANGED MY LIFE! It helped me lose 35 lbs. and reversed my chronic disease in the process. I promise if I can do it, YOU CAN TOO! You can forget about food restriction, enjoy food once again, and live life to the fullest!

Chapter 3: Modern Weight Loss Myths: Creating Confusion Since the Early 1900s.

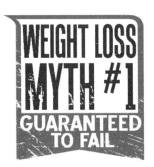

Losing weight is all about Calorie Intake

The term "calorie" was brought to America by a scientist named Wilbur O. Atwater in 1887. A calorie was defined as "the amount of energy required to increase the temperature of 1 kilogram of water by 1 degree Kelvin." By using thermometers, hygrometers, electric condensers, pumps, and fans, Atwater found he could precisely measure the exchange of heat, air, and matter. Initially, the measuring of calories was used in applications of engineering & physics ONLY. In later years, other scientists also heated fat, protein, carbs, and sugar and found out the calorie content of those as well. Logging our calorie intake became officially popular in 1918 when Lulu Hunt Peters published her bestselling book, Diet & Health. She presented counting calories as the key to maintaining weight.

What everybody seems to forget is that food is SO much more than calories! When you ingest a food, whether it is a hamburger, a popsicle, or a whole-wheat brownie – each has many possible uses for the body. Depending on the food you eat (and the quality of it), your body may use it to build & repair tissues, make enzymes, make hormones, produce bile or stomach acid, store it for future energy in the form of glycogen or fat, or it may fail to be digested and become only partially absorbed, harming your delicate gut bacteria.

Calories are NOT considered equal in the body. It is the *quality* of your calorie that matters.

The calorie theory, also known as the "eat less, move more" theory, is eternally flawed because it ignores the importance of nutrients – **the very reason why we eat food in the first place!** When you focus on calorie restriction, you lose out on vital nutrients, vitamins, and minerals.

"What you eat makes quite a difference. Just counting calories won't matter much unless you look at the kinds of calories you're eating."

-Dr. Dariush Mozaffarian

2 tootsie rolls
70 calories

VS.

1 egg
70 calories

Ingredients: sugar, corn syrup, partially hydrogenated soybean condensed skim milk, cocoa, whey lethicin, and natural & artificial flavors. No essential nutrients or minerals.

Full of fat-soluble vitamins A, D, & E, as well as B1, B2, B6 & B12, one egg packs a powerhouse of nutrients. Additionally, it provides Folate And the minerals Phosphorous Calcium, Iron, Iodine, Selenium & Zinc. as well as antioxidants lutein & zeaxanthin.

The truth is, the conventional wisdom about why we get fat is simply wrong. It's not about energy balance; it's not about "overconsumption of calories" or "taking in more calories than we burn." It's about something else entirely: how the human body regulates fat metabolism and the accumulation of fat in our adipose tissue.

-Gary Taubes

What you need to understand is when you reduce your calorie intake, **your body interprets it as starvation** – a highly stressful situation. And what do our bodies produce when we are stressed? The hormone cortisol. Chronic high levels of cortisol in the blood leads to immune suppression, fatigue, reduced thyroid & metabolic function, and last but not least – fat storage. Counting and reducing calories is a one way ticket to an inefficient metabolism and ultimate weight gain.

A study published in 2012 by the Journal of American Medical Association found that weight loss from a reduced-calorie diet resulted in a significantly slower metabolism, and contributed to a faster re-gain of lost weight.

"The only people successful at permanently reducing calorie intake by at least half are those that develop an eating disorder, the deadliest known psychological disease, which affects 11 million Americans, mostly young women."

-Matt Stone, Diet Recovery.

I'm proud to say I have never once counted my calorie intake. For that, I am grateful! Because calories are not created equal, because we are more than just machines burning fuel, we can forget about our calorie intake. Let's focus on nutrition! Look for foods that are satisfying and nourishing.

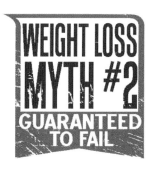

Exercise is necessary for weight loss

"Be sure to get your 45 min. of cardio a day!" "Work your core!" "Feel the burn!" We encounter these exercise taglines numerous times each day. Each grocery store checkout line, magazine article at the doctor's office, and numerous internet sites all claim to have the secret trick to the ultimate body. The catch? It involves spending hours at the gym. Do you think losing weight really involves hitting the gym every day for the REST OF YOUR LIFE?

What if I told you that numerous studies say NO? The most recent study debunking the exercise myth was published in 2013. Researchers analyzed data from 33,060 runners and 15,045 walkers over six years. What did they find? They found that moderate intensity and vigorous intensity running produced similar results.

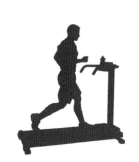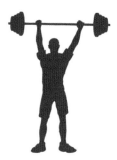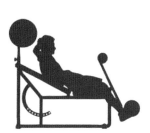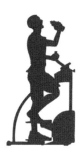

The idea that we have to exercise like crazy to lose weight is FALSE. If I lost weight with absolutely 0:00 minutes of exercise, you can do it with light exercise or none at all. You don't have to be a boot camp graduate to be successful in losing weight. Our ancestors would literally laugh their butts off if they saw us running on the treadmill or lifting weights. We *can maintain* our weight with healthy eating and moderate activity, believe you me!

Some people really, truly love to exercise hardcore – and I'm not here to slam those people. "Whatever floats your boat," my Dad always said. But for the rest of us, let's be honest here. Do you really LOVE to run on a treadmill for 45 minutes a day & lift weights in your spare time?

Yeah, I didn't think so. Me neither.

Our bodies were designed to move, but not designed to exercise excessively, a habit that can lead to chronic stress on the body.

"Aggressive physical training cannot change fundamental mobility and stability problems at an effective rate without also introducing a degree of compensation and increased risk of injury...We should train muscles in the way we use them."

-Gray Cook, <u>Movement</u>

Moderate activity, similar to our ancestor's daily lives, can supply enough exercise our bodies need. Simple activities like riding a bike, yoga/stretching, weeding your garden, walking, and even playing with your children can give your body the movement it needs, and the enjoyment you feel supports healthy brain function! Stress-inducing high intensity exercising, on the other hand, has the opposite effect.

"For example, if you jog for a couple of hours every day, this is said to raise your metabolism because you are burning more calories through exercise. This is false. Jogging typically lowers metabolism, especially when taken to excess – instead it is the Total Energy Expenditure or TEE that is raised by burning more calories through exercise while the basal metabolic rate or BMR typically drops. If you stop jogging, it is easier to gain fat than ever before because your metabolism has been lowered by this form of exercise. This is just one of the many myths surrounding metabolism."

-Matt Stone, <u>Diet Recovery</u>

Is your exercise causing your body stress or enjoyment? If any exercise is stressful and you don't find any enjoyment in it, you should probably rethink that choice. Exercise is wonderful for training our muscles and cardiovascular system and is a necessary part of balanced health, but be sure to remember that if your focus is to burn calories in the hopes of losing weight, you're fighting a losing battle.

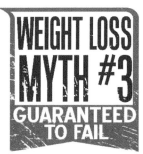

WEIGHT LOSS MYTH #3 GUARANTEED TO FAIL

Get your lean protein here, get your lean protein there, be sure to get it everywhere!

Honestly, I get so very tired of people saying, "Be sure to get your protein!" Or "Eat lots of lean meats to stay full!" While protein does play an important part in a healthy & balanced diet, the statement that we need a lot of it (and the lean versions) to stay full and lose weight has been overemphasized.

The problem with LEAN PROTEIN is when you remove the fat from the protein, you make it hard for the body to absorb. Protein simply cannot be utilized by the body without the aid of fats. Isn't it amazing that the highest sources of protein that exist are naturally full of fat-soluble vitamins? Eggs, Whole Milk, Fish, Meat, and Nuts -- these all are accompanied by one or more of the fat-soluble vitamins A, D, E, or K2, which are needed for the absorption of protein! Beans are often proclaimed by plant-based eaters to be a great source of protein. However, many people don't realize that beans are primarily full of carbohydrates. This is why traditional societies would always cook beans with a ham bone or pork fat to increase the digestibility of it!

Ultimately, consumption of low-fat dairy, lean meats, and egg whites can result in a deficiency of those precious fat-soluble vitamins. Many people mistakenly believe the Japanese eat a low-fat diet and even more people refer to the Japanese as a culture who has the longest life expectancy. While it is true that the Japanese do have the longest life span of any nation, it is false that they live a low-fat lifestyle. The Japanese regularly consume eggs, pork, beef, chicken, and seafood. They do not eat lean, skinless, boneless versions of these, but rather, the full-fat and vitamin rich versions.

In lean protein, you've essentially taken a source of protein, like meat or eggs, and removed the fat. Now you are left with egg whites and skinless, boneless chicken breasts. You have effectively turned a most natural & nutritious food into an unnatural and incomplete one. And on top of that, you lose the satisfying flavor! Don't you want your food to be delicious and savory? I promise you it is possible to ENJOY your fatty food and LOSE WEIGHT!

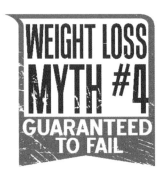
WEIGHT LOSS MYTH #4 GUARANTEED TO FAIL

A low-fat diet will make you skinny!

I want you to repeat this sentence – Fat, yes even saturated fat, is an amazing, wonderful thing that every single body needs. I'll admit it; fat is something I used to avoid. I really wanted to lose weight and so I ignorantly listened to all the advice plastered over magazines, TV shows, and internet. Low-fat seemed like the only answer to true health.

In the 1950s, Ancel Keys, an American scientist, had an interest in the human diet and its relationship to cardiovascular disease. His research led to a study known as the Seven Countries Study. After observing individuals who lived over 100 years, Keys concluded that a diet high in animal fats contributed to heart disease. As a result of his findings, he theorized that animal fats contributed to weight gain and disease. His "lipid hypothesis" became known to the world when, in 1956, representatives of the American Heart Association appeared on television to announce a healthy diet meant a low-fat one. Dr. Dudley White (who also happened to be President Eisenhower's physician) disagreed with Key's "lipid hypothesis" and pointed out the correlation between the consumption of processed vegetable oils and increase of heart attacks. After all, the use of margarine had quadrupled, while egg consumption had declined by half. Coconut oil had been replaced with vegetable oil, and lard had been replaced with hydrogenated Crisco. Yet, traditional fats found in eggs, butter, cream, and animal meats were touted by the American Heart Association as unhealthy and a "heart attack just waiting to happen."

The truth is that fats from animals **AND** some plant sources work together and provide the building blocks for our body, give us energy, and help us feel full longer. We are often told that cholesterol is bad, but it plays an important role in the body. The "lipid hypothesis," also known as the cholesterol myth, was just a really bad guess by doctors in the 1920s and has been debunked over and over again!

The fact that the early testing of the "lipid hypothesis" was performed on rabbits, who are **HERBIVORES**, should be reason enough to show that this theory was wrong. I'm not a scientist, but I'm pretty sure when you feed an herbivore (animal who can only digest plants) gobs of animal fat, it prolly will die. Prolly.

What's more incredulous is that Ancel Keys, the scientist who first theorized that cholesterol caused heart disease, yes the very man who started this whole fear of fat, **later changed his stance on cholesterol and its relationship to heart disease.**

"The evidence—both from experiments and from field surveys—indicates that the cholesterol content, per se, of all natural diets has NO significant effect on either the serum cholesterol level or the development of atherosclerosis in man."

-Ancel Keys,
The relationship of the diet to the development of atherosclerosis in man.

Need more proof? A recent study found that over half of patients admitted for heart attacks have perfectly normal levels of cholesterol! The "lipid hypothesis" has never been proven because the truth is that cholesterol is a poor indicator of heart disease. Isn't it interesting how the countries of Japan, Austria, and Greece – all tied for longevity - eat high fat diets? The Japanese eat high amounts of beef, chicken, pork, fish, and eggs – all of which have significant amounts of saturated fat. The French, who also consume a high-fat diet, have a lower rate of heart disease than Americans. Why? It's because contrary to popular Western belief, fat does a body good! In the well-known Lyon Diet Heart study performed by French Researchers in the 1990s, they found that levels of cholesterol didn't change between those eating a high-fat diet and a low-fat diet, and, in fact, they saw a 76% reduction in heart-related deaths in the high-fat group!

Cholesterol has many important jobs in your body. It helps regulate hormones & stress, thereby reducing one's risk of cancer & heart disease. Also, because the brain is largely composed of fat, higher cholesterol levels also increase serotonin function. Serotonin is the body's "feel good" chemical and plays an important role in our mental health. Fat helps maintain the wall of the intestines, preventing leaky gut syndrome. The liver needs cholesterol to create bile, which is vital for digestion & the assimilation of fat.

"Cholesterol is an essential molecule without which there would be no life, so important that virtually every cell in the body is capable of synthesizing it."

Stephen Sinatra & Jonny Bowden, The Great Cholesterol Myth

So why are we still so confused about cholesterol? Why are we told at every corner to eat low-fat and fear those blood cholesterol levels? As much as I like to avoid being a conspiracy theorist, I have to point out that the cholesterol-lowering drugs (statins) bring in a whopping 30 BILLION dollars per year for the drug-making companies. And on top of that, when the "acceptable" cholesterol numbers were lowered in 2004, EIGHT out of NINE members of the National Cholesterol Education Program, who "set" that official number, had financial ties to the pharmaceutical industry. This means that the people, who are telling us our cholesterol numbers are too high, are the very people who make money if we take cholesterol-lowering drugs!

Now if that's not shocking, I don't know what is.

Mary Enig, Ph.D, one of the top lipid biochemists in the country, points out in her book, Eat Fat, Lose Fat, that when Americans were eating whole fat foods such as cream, butter, grass-fed meats, and raw milk, heart disease was lower than ever.

She also writes,

> *"As the French maintain their trim physiques while consuming triple cream brie, steak au poivre, and béarnaise sauce, most American adults would barely dare to drink a glass of whole-fat milk."*

Have you ever wondered why it is so hard to lose weight and stick to a diet? What if I told you that eating low-fat is the main reason you have had trouble losing that weight? When you remove the fat-soluble vitamins from your diet, the ones that aid in digestion, make you feel nourished, and signal to your brain that you are full, you are ultimately left feeling hungry & deprived.

> *"In fact, even a simple drop in body fat levels due to inadequate calorie intake lowers the hormone leptin – the master hormone well-understood to regulate appetite, metabolism, and immune system potency. It also raises the stress hormone cortisol, the primary aging and immunosuppressive hormone."*
>
> *- Matt Stone, Diet Recovery*

You don't need willpower to lose weight; you just need more real food fats!

So which fat is good & which is bad? The most important thing for you to remember about fat is that it's just like any other food...you must find it in its most natural & healthy form. If you have Crisco, Canola, or Vegetable oil in your pantry...it's time to GET. THEM. OUT! These oils are nothing more than highly processed, hydrogenated garbage. Your body does not even recognize them, and, in fact, your body creates inflammation just to get rid of them. So please, remove them from your diet and embrace REAL FATS like butter, lard, tallow, and other animal fats, as well as olive oil & coconut oil!

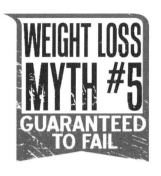

Watch those carbs, they are evil!

Somewhere around the time when sugar was found to raise insulin levels dangerously high in diabetics, scientists came to the conclusion that **all carbohydrates**, once broken down into glucose, had the possibility of creating an insulin surge in any body – diabetic or otherwise. The truth is our bodies need carbohydrates to function at an optimal level. When a carb is broken down into glucose, it has many uses in the body. Whether your body uses it for energy, repairs, growth, hormone regulation, or muscle movement, you can trust that your body definitely needs it!

It's when we try to limit our carbohydrate intake that things start to really get messed up!

When we reduce our carb intake our body is all, "Wha???" and then it shrugs its shoulders and decides to do whatever it can to make glucose. First, it uses our fat cells to try to create some glucose, also known as lipolysis. When that doesn't work, the body gets creative and starts using any tissue from the body to create its precious energy source. This is referred to as gluconeogenesis. Now things start to get really juicy…

The human body is AMAZING at compensation. The problem is, compensation is a lot like telling a white lie. Eventually it leads to another white lie…and another white lie…and another, until the whole thing goes kaput.

Prolonged restriction of carbohydrates produces a "stressed" situation in our bodies. As a result, adrenaline & cortisol (the stress hormones) are released. This is why at first you feel amazing and lose weight on a low carb diet! You're all, "Woo-hoo! I'm rockin' this new diet!" and your body's all, "Wow, I am burnt out. Where's my fuel? Oh well, let's just make our own – bring out the adrenaline & cortisol again."

The human body was NOT designed to live in a stressful state for extended periods of time.

When you finally give in and eat carbs again (because trust me, you will), unfortunately, your body is not doin' so well. By now, you will notice you are getting sick a lot, experiencing digestive issues, low libido, and generally just feeling crappy. Congratulations! You've successfully screwed up your metabolism and all of its functions!

But don't worry, there's a way to get back to health – and yes, it involves eating carbs. Lucky for you, carbs are not the enemy anymore. Did our ancestors eat carbs?

Yes! Did they maintain a healthy & natural weight? Yes! Did they have diabetes? No!

> *"In ideal conditions, your body should have access to all three macronutrient (carbohydrates, fat and protein) in relatively balanced amounts. Sure, your body is technically capable of making its own fuel if needed, but this is a sort of emergency back-up plan for when the right balance of fuel isn't coming from your diet. If you want to stress out your metabolism, start denying it some of the most basic elements it needs to survive."*
>
> *-Elizabeth Walling*, <u>The Nourished Metabolism</u>

ARE ALL CARBS CREATED EQUALLY?

There are two kinds of carbohydrates – simple & complex. The difference between the two is their molecular structure. Simple carbs are closer to the molecular structure of glucose and are readily usable by the body. Complex carbs are a little more, well, complex and contain a long chain of molecules that the body has to first break down before using.

Fruit contains FRUCTOSE, a simple carbohydrate. When a fruit is juiced and only the sugar (fructose) is extracted, it can produce a significant spike in blood sugar. BUT in its **whole form,** coupled with vitamins, nutrients, minerals, and fiber, FRUCTOSE won't nearly have the same detriment. When you eat an apple, you are eating a whole, perfect food, and your body does not experience such a high spike in blood sugar & insulin levels. When you drink apple juice, you are drinking pure FRUCTOSE, a simple carbohydrate, and if you drank it every single day, over time, yes, it would have a harmful effect on your body. The same goes for highly processed sugars found in processed foods & soda drinks. These have a negative effect on the body because of the incredible spike in blood sugar they cause when ingested.

The awesome benefit of eating real food is that you really don't have to worry about counting carbs. If you are focusing on mainly whole & real food, including {properly prepared} whole grains, fruits, root vegetables, and unrefined sweeteners, you shouldn't have any problems. And the world won't end when you occasionally eat a simple carbohydrate such as white flour, white rice, or fruit juice because they won't be part of your regular diet.

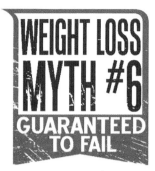

Control those Portions!
Eat 6 Small Meals a day!
Don't eat past 7pm!
Drink your weight in water!

For my last weight loss myth, I decided to group together the most common rules that seem to be added onto every diet plan. Let's debunk these one by one...

Portion Control

The main idea behind portion control is to control our intake of food, am I right? Many people argue that without portion control, we are gluttonous overeaters with no way of stopping. Have you ever wondered why people overeat in the first place? Oh sure, some people say it's because of the addicting power of sugar & some say it stems from emotional issues. Wanna know the real reason people overeat?

It's because they are **STARVING!** Yesiree. Those who eat a Standard American Diet are the most overweight but also the most malnourished people on the planet! Our bodies are begging for real food – for those precious nutrients, vitamins, and minerals. Our bodies are begging for **NOURISHMENT!** I'm gonna tell you a little secret. I live on the wild side and don't use portion control. Are you shocked? Wanna know how I stay thin without portion control? It's simple. I eat nutrient-dense real food, and eat until I feel satisfied. Remember when we talked about how all calories are NOT created equally?

Leptin – the hormone that tells our brain we're full – floods our bloodstream while we're eating. But guess what? **Leptin is deactivated when we eat high amounts of fake processed foods**. Remember when you ate that whole pan of rice krispie bars? Yeah, probably not the best idea.

The good news is that we can get that hormone Leptin to start working again! All it takes is eating real, nutrient-rich whole foods to get that signal back on course. And then next time when you are enjoying a pot roast, buttery mashed potatoes with gravy, and a side of green beans, you can feel satisfied and stop when YOU feel nourished.

Bottom line: Become an intuitive eater by listening to your body's biofeedback. Eat enough to feel satisfied and trust in your body's instincts.

Eat 6 Small Meals a Day

While I'm all about eating as much as you want, when you want – **also known as eating when you're hungry** – I want to debunk the myth that our bodies somehow become more efficient when we eat small meals all day long.

Unlike animals such as horses, cows, and sheep, the human digestive system doesn't do well with grazing. Because our stomach has many important tasks – secreting gastric juices, churning and mixing our food, and opening and closing the valves that lead to the intestines -- our bodies need a significant rest between meals. Since our digestion also relies on secretions from the pancreas and liver, we can conclude that our entire body enjoys a good rest between meals. Frequent snacking and the common "eat 6 small meals a day" approach will eventually lead to an exhausted digestive system and produce a variety of symptoms such as indigestion, heartburn, bloating, and gas.

Carbohydrates, proteins, and fats all stay in the stomach for different periods of time, so in order to have optimal nourishment and satisfaction, simply eat a balanced meal without food restriction of any main nutrients and you'll be set! The exception would be if you are genuinely hungry between meals. As you transition from a Standard American Diet to a nourishing one, your malnourished body will typically eat more between meals. This is partly due to the hormone leptin being suppressed for many years, and the weak metabolism that needs calories to heal.

Bottom line: Eat when you're hungry. Eat nourishing foods. But don't feel the pressure to snack all day long.

Don't Eat Past 7pm

While it is true that our body's metabolic rate slows down as we get closer to bedtime, if you're coming from a poor diet, understandably your body will be craving real food nourishment. You're also learning how to eat intuitively – a practice that you probably haven't implemented for years. Listen to your body's bio feedback. If you are hungry at 7, 8, 9, or even 10 pm at night, then by all means EAT SOMETHING!

If you are eating a nutrient-dense diet consisting of real food, your body will feel nourished and you no longer need to worry about these silly rules.

Bottom line: Trust in your instincts. If you are hungry, then EAT!

Drink your weight in water!

The pressure to drink gallons of water is at an all-time high, and believe me, I've fallen for the hype myself. But contrary to popular belief, drinking 8 glasses of water a day is not the standard for everyone. In fact, it's quite the opposite. When you drink too much water and ignore those warning signs – excessive urination, brain fog, and cold hands – you are setting up your body for a host of problems.

One of the first things I learned in nursing school is how to start IV's. When a patient is admitted to the hospital, whether deathly sick or sick with the stomach flu, the protocol is to start an IV and administer a solution to **HYDRATE** them. Do we start IV's and administer **PURE WATER?** Absolutely not! That would dilute their electrolytes so fast it would kill them. IV hydration is done with either a saline solution or a saline solution with additional potassium & glucose (sugar). This is because the extracellular fluid inside our bodies is not 100% water, but a mixture of many minerals like calcium, sodium, potassium, as well as a small amount of glucose. We need this to balance our pH and basically stay alive. We are taught that over-hydration is impossible, but it's simply not true. Over-hydration can lead to electrolyte imbalance, headaches, muscle spasms, insomnia, fatigue, low body temperature, suppressed metabolism, and WEIGHT GAIN. The body is great at regulation. When our bodies need more food, we feel hungry. When our bodies need more water, we feel thirsty.

I used to drink a gallon of water a day, because, well, I thought it was "healthy." The first thing I would do in the morning was chug a big 'ol quart of water. Bleh. I hated it. It made me feel nauseous. And cold. And foggy-headed. But I did it because I thought it was the "healthy" thing to do. Talk about not being in touch with my body. Now, I simply don't drink pure water unless I am thirsty. Other than that, I get my REAL hydration from fruits & vegetables, as well as other fluids I drink like raw milk, fermented drinks like water kefir or kombucha, and homemade Gatorade. I don't try to meet some water intake quota. I simply drink when I am thirsty.

"But I've heard when we are thirsty that means we are already dehydrated!"

Seriously? Are we really on the brink of dehydration when our body finally tells us it needs water? If that were true, then when our body tells us we are hungry, we must be seconds away from death from starvation! Just like our body knows when it needs to blink, breathe, sleep, and poop, it knows when it needs hydration. And thirst is the preferred method of communication.

"Overhydration [and overdilution of extracellular fluid] is MUCH more common in the water-loving, dehydration-panicked, salt-phobic realm of the modern internet-scouring health nerd, and the symptoms of overhydration/dilution trump that of being mildly

dehydrated by a long shot – typically existing on a near constant basis and creating suffering daily at one or more points during the day.

Forcing yourself to meet some quota of fluids, drinking because you think you should, having a hot beverage because you are cold – this is very powerfully depleting and can trigger some real health problems in someone in a compromised metabolic condition."

– *Matt Stone,* <u>Eat for Heat</u>

How much water do I drink? In the mornings, I drink milk and typically have fruit with my breakfast, and through that I am obtaining water. After my morning farm chores, I usually drink a glass or two of water, and then also have fruit & vegetables, and typically some kombucha for lunch, which is another source of fluids. In the evening, I drink a couple glasses of water again. I try to focus on eating real food and drinking only when I am thirsty.

<u>Bottom line: Drink water when you are thirsty, not just because it is "healthy."</u>

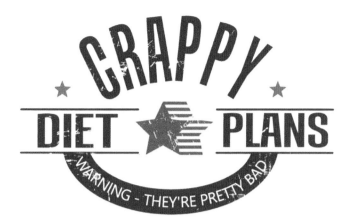

Just so we are clear on what we have learned about all the diet myths out there, let's go over the crappy diet plans that promote these failed concepts. **Each one of these diets promotes a restriction of one of the key nutrients – carbs, protein, or fat.** Often they promote a restriction of calories as well. Do you see a running theme here? That's right folks, we just keep wasting our time, trying to demonize one of the 3 main nutrients. Can we just please chillax?! Carbohydrates, Proteins, and Fats all play major roles in our health, and we need to stop following **FADS** and **JUST EAT REAL FOOD!**

- **Nutrisystem** – Low-calorie, low-fat. Sells processed food.
- **Weight Watchers** – Low-calorie, low-fat. Promotes processed food.
- **Jenny Craig** – Low-calorie, low-fat. Sells processed food.
- **The Zone** – Low-carb, low-fat.
- The Atkins Diet – Low-carb.
- **The South Beach Diet** – Low-calorie, low-carb, low-fat.
- **The HCG Diet** – Low-calorie, low-carb, low-fat.
- The Glycemic Index Diet – Low-carb, low-fat.
- **The Blood Type Diet** – Low-carb, low-fat, or low-protein depending on your blood type.
- **The Acid/Alkaline Diet** – Low-protein, low-fat.
- **Ornish Diet** – Low-fat, low-protein.
Vegan or strict plant-based diets – Low-fat, low-protein.

I'm tired of researching crappy diets, so I'll stop now. But you're probably asking one question. If these diets are so bad, then why do they work for some people? The answer, my friends, is that when you restrict a basic nutrient, or even overall calories, your body goes into stress mode. You are losing weight because adrenaline & cortisol are pumping through your veins and using up energy. AND this is the **EXACT** reason why most people gain it all back after coming off these diets. By then, your metabolism is shot and lower than ever and is just itching to pack on the pounds as recovery from that awful diet.

Chapter 4: Vegan, Vegetarian, & Plant-Based Diets

For a while, after my "internet nutrition education," I was wrongly convinced that I needed to eat a plant-based diet to be successful in my weight loss & reversal of disease. Let's go over the spectrum of plant-based dieters, because it can get confusing ya'll.

Vegetarians typically eat no meat, but may still include dairy and eggs in their diet, calling themselves **lacto-ovo-vegetarians.** Those who also include seafood in their diet are called **pescetarians.**

Plant-based dieters typically eat very little animal products, and many eat none at all.

Vegans strictly avoid all animal products including meat, dairy, eggs, fish, and honey.

Raw Food Vegans exclude all animal products and focus on a diet of all raw foods, mainly fruits and vegetables with some seeds/nuts/grains that have been sprouted or grown into grass.

Are humans supposed to be herbivores (plant-eaters), carnivores (meat-eaters), or omnivores (plant & meat eaters)?

The basic argument of plant-based eaters is that our bodies are designed to eat only plants. Animal products should be eaten very rarely, if ever. They show pictures of gorillas and assume if a gorilla could build massive muscles from eating plants, then we, who are similar in structure to primates, must be designed to eat only plants as well.

There are many flaws in this theory. First of all, gorillas do not eat only fruits & vegetables. Gorillas eat plants AND bugs AND eggs they find in the wild. Second, gorillas have the smallest brains yet the largest digestive tracts of primates. We, as humans, are opposite. We have larger, complex brains (that need fats), and a smaller digestive tract. Third, and most importantly, is that gorillas, zebras, giraffes, elephants, hippos, rhinos, horses, cows, sheep, and goats all have one thing we humans do not.

They produce the bacteria needed to digest CELLULOSE (also known as fiber). Cellulose is in every plant. Plant-eating animals (also known as herbivores) CAN break down cellulose. We, as humans, cannot. This is why when you eat corn, you'll notice some, ahem, undigested bits. Plants (and the cellulose they contain) act very differently in our bodies than in herbivorous animals. For them, it is a primary source of nutrition. For us, it is a small amount of nutrition and mostly roughage or fiber. The indigestible fiber in plants helps add bulk to our poop, for the sole reason that it runs right through us. Plants can provide many good vitamins & minerals. But when we try to obtain **all** of our nutrition from plants, it eventually leads to deficiencies.

Are plant-only diets nutritionally superior or deficient?

Some promote these diets as healthier because of the avoidance or low consumption of animal foods. Many claim if you don't eat animal products, you won't get heart disease or cancer. **This is simply not true.** Vegetarians, vegans, and plant-based dieters all can get cancer, and some types of cancers are more prevalent in people that eat these diets. Steve Jobs, a Raw Food Vegan who ate primarily fruit & fruit juice, developed pancreatic cancer. High amounts of fruit sugar (fructose) found in fruits & fruit juices can cause stress to the pancreas, whose job it is to regulate blood sugar by secreting insulin. Robin Gibb of the Bee Gees, another famous vegan, died of colon cancer at the age of 62. In fact, colon cancer is high among vegans, and recent studies have linked a low consumption of B12 (found only in animal products) to colon cancer. Michael Clarke Duncan, an actor well known for his role in The Green Mile, died at age 55 of a heart attack. He was a long-time vegan and spokesman for the animal activist group, PETA.

While there are many, many benefits to eating fruits & vegetables, **a complete avoidance of animal foods** will eventually lead to deficiencies. A plant-based diet is missing complete proteins (all 9 amino acids), fat-soluble vitamins such as A, D, E, & K2, minerals such as iron & zinc, and B12.

Some vegans will argue that although plant foods are missing complete proteins, they need only eat a variety of plant foods every day to ensure their diet contains all 9 amino acids. However, the absorption of plant protein is hindered because plant foods are conveniently wrapped in, you guessed it, cellulose. Yep, plenty of indigestible fiber to keep your body from absorbing that protein.

Another argument of vegans is that plants contain fat-soluble vitamins as well. This is only partly true. Let's break 'em down:

Vitamin A

What it does: A vital nutrient, Vitamin A is essential for eyesight, needed for the growth & repair of bones & tissues, aids in the digestion of protein, and promotes a healthy immune system by providing healthy mucus in the lungs, skin, and mouth. Deficiencies in Vitamin A can produce blindness, stunted growth, and frequent infections, and are associated with a high infant mortality rate.

How to get it: There is no plant source of Vitamin A. There is only proto-vitamin

A, also called beta-carotene. When you eat beta-carotene, your body must convert it to Vitamin A before it can be used. In developing countries where the diet is primarily plant-based, Vitamin A deficiency is a serious problem. Children and the elderly have particular trouble with this conversion from beta-carotene to Vitamin A.

> *"Diabetics and those with poor thyroid function, a group that could well include at least half the adult US population, cannot make the conversion. Children make the conversion very poorly and infants not at all — they must obtain their precious stores of vitamin A from animal fats— yet the low-fat diet is often recommended for children. Strenuous physical exercise, excessive consumption of alcohol, excessive consumption of iron (especially from "fortified" white flour and breakfast cereal), use of a number of popular drugs, excessive consumption of polyunsaturated fatty acids, zinc deficiency and even cold weather can hinder the conversion of carotenes to vitamin A, as does the low-fat diet."*
>
> *-Sally A. Fallon & Mary G. Enig, The Vitamin A Saga*

Ironically, the conversion only works when a plant-based beta-carotene is combined with animal fat.

> *"Carotenes are converted by the action of bile salts, and very little bile reaches the intestine when a meal is low in fat. The epicure who puts butter on his vegetables and adds cream to his vegetable soup is wiser than he knows. Butterfat stimulates the secretion of bile needed to convert carotenes from vegetables into vitamin A, and at the same time supplies very easily absorbed true vitamin A."*
>
> *-Sally A. Fallon & Mary G. Enig, The Vitamin A Saga*

Vitamin D

What it does: Vitamin D supports bone health. Calcium simply cannot be used by the body without the aid of Vitamin D. Vitamin D will also aid in the removal of harmful toxic metals such as cadmium, aluminum, and strontium. Probably one of the most important tasks of Vitamin D is hormone production & regulation. Problems with your adrenals (which can be manifested through **fibromyalgia)**, problems with your thyroid (which can be manifested through **hypothyroidism)**, and problems with your sex hormones (which can be manifested through **infertility)** can all be related to a deficiency in fat-soluble Vitamin D.

How to get it: There are no plant based sources of Vitamin D, with the exception of UV-irradiated mushrooms, a modern process attempting to mimic what animal foods & the sun provide for us naturally. Unfortunately, UV-irradiated mushrooms only supply 21 IU of Vitamin D per mushroom. To obtain your daily requirement of Vitamin D, you'd have to eat 50 mushrooms per day! One tablespoon of lard obtained from naturally foraged pigs (like our ancestors have been eating for thousands of years) contains 1500 IU! Other food sources of Vitamin D are egg yolks, cod liver oil, cold water oily fish, oysters, and caviar or roe.

When you are attempting to obtain your Vitamin D from the sun, first you must understand that the sun distributes 3 different rays, and UV-B is the only ray that stimulates our bodies to produce Vitamin D. Most people don't know that UV-B is only present at mid-day hours at higher latitudes. I didn't say altitude, I said latitude. So depending on where you live, you may not be obtaining very much Vitamin D from the sun at all. Even if you live at high latitudes, for your body to make Vitamin D from the sun you must be outside from 10am-2pm only, as the other hours of the day will supply a higher amount of UV-A rays, and **you will become sunburned long before you can get those crucial UV-B rays & Vitamin D.** Animals are immune to UV-A rays, and therefore aren't able to become sunburned. They are superheroes at synthesizing Vitamin D. I'm not saying we can't get Vitamin D from the sun, but for some people it might be difficult, and Vitamin D deficiency is a common ailment today. You still obtain some Vitamin D from the sun, but not the full amount you need.

While the current daily recommendation of Vitamin D is only 400-800 IU, Dr. Weston A. Price (remember him? He's the one who traveled the world and researched vibrantly healthy societies.) noticed that traditional cultures ate 8-10 times that amount, around 4,000 IU per day. Today, Vitamin-D therapy is currently being used to treat cancer, osteoporosis, heart disease, hormonal problems, and depression.

Vitamin E

What it does: Vitamin E is vital for cell health and protects your skin & circulatory system. It is also a powerful anti-oxidant.

How to get it: There are **both** animal & plant sources of Vitamin E. Butter and Liver from primarily grass-fed animals and wild salmon roe are great sources, as well as raw almonds and raw hazelnuts.

"The absence of whole grains and liver, traditional foods rich in vitamin E, from the modern diet has resulted in widespread deficiencies. Much evidence demonstrates this has significantly contributed to the modern epidemic of heart disease and other problems."

-*Ron Schmid*, <u>Traditional Foods Are Your Best Medicine</u>

Plant-based dieters must take care to properly prepare their grains, nuts, and seeds by soaking, sprouting, or sour leavening in order to unlock Vitamin E and other nutrients from these foods.

Vitamin K

What it does: Many people are not aware that Vitamin K is divided into 2 separate vitamins – K1 & K2. K1 exists in the chlorophyll of green plants. When it is consumed, the body uses K1 for blood clotting and then converts the rest of the K1 to K2.

Studies on rats have shown that it's harder than we thought for the body to completely convert Vitamin K1 into Vitamin K2, suggesting that relying on plants as our only source of Vitamin K is not going to help us much when we need K2.

That's why we need animal sources of K2, arguably one of the MOST IMPORTANT fat-soluble vitamins. One of Vitamin K2's VERY important jobs is to regulate calcium. It tells the body to place calcium in the correct places in our body; for example, in our bones & teeth. It also tells the body where to NOT deposit calcium; for example, in our arteries, kidneys, and joints. K2's job of regulating mineral absorption CANNOT be understated. Your bones and teeth rely on Vitamin K2 to maintain correct mineral levels. Deficiencies in Vitamin K2 will result in bone loss & fractures, dental caries (cavities), and discolored teeth. Osteoporosis and heart disease have been linked with low levels of K2.

How to get it: While Vitamin K1 resides in rapidly growing green plants such as spinach, swiss chard, kale, and broccoli, your body must convert part of it to Vitamin K2, and like we talked about before, the human body does not do this well with raw veggies eaten alone. What's more, **the absorption of Vitamin K1 and your body's ability to convert it to K2 is greatly improved if it's eaten with butter or oil.** Creamed spinach, anyone? Animal sources of Vitamin K2, ready for the body to absorb, are goose liver pate, hard cheeses such as gouda, soft cheeses such as brie, egg yolks, butter, chicken, beef, bacon, and whole milk. Natto (fermented soybeans) and homemade fermented foods, such as sauerkraut, are great plant sources of Vitamin K2.

"A study recently published by the European Prospective Investigation into Cancer and Nutrition (EPIC) has revealed that increased intake of vitamin K2 may reduce the risk of prostate cancer by 35 percent. The authors point out that the benefits of K2 were most pronounced for advanced prostate cancer, and, importantly, that vitamin K1 did not offer any prostate benefits. The findings were based on data from more than 11,000 men taking part in the EPIC Heidelberg cohort. It adds to a small but fast-growing body

of science supporting the potential health benefits of vitamin K2 for bone, cardiovascular, skin, brain, and now prostate health."

- *Chris Kesser, Vitamin K2:* <u>The Missing Nutrient</u>
-

Zinc

Plant-based dieters are frequently low in zinc, an important cofactor for enzymes. This is because although zinc is found in grains, legumes, fruits, and vegetables, they contain much lower amounts than animal sources.

Also, plants contain compounds such as phytates, oxalates, polyphenols, and fiber that inhibit the absorption of zinc. Animal sources like seafood & beef contain up to 24 times the amount of zinc than plant based foods.

Iron

Iron is found in eggs, fish, liver, meat & some green leafy vegetables, but just like zinc, iron from animal sources is more easily absorbed than that from plant sources. Additionally, iron-fortified packaged foods are inorganic in nature and are completely unusable by the body. In fact, high amounts of inorganic iron from iron-fortified packaged foods are considered by the body as a toxin and have been linked to heart disease & cancer.

B12

B12 is exclusively found in animal foods and is vital for brain & nervous system function as well as healthy red blood cells. In order to not become deficient, a plant-based dieter must eat animal foods or take a supplement to obtain Vitamin B12. Nutritional yeast is often thought by vegans to be a good source of Vitamin B12. The truth is, however, that nutritional yeast does not naturally contain B12 and is instead fortified with a synthetic form. A fortified, packaged product can never do as well for our bodies as what is found in nature. A recent study found that 46% of lacto-ovo vegetarians and 64% of vegans are deficient in B12. Proof that nothing in a factory works as well as what comes naturally.

The SOY Saga:

When I say "soy," the first thing you probably think of is "healthy." **This literally couldn't be further from the truth!** Plant-based dieters typically rely on soy products as a substitute for meat. They eat tofu and proclaim it as a "heart-healthy" choice. Many people think that soy is healthy because it is often used in Asian dishes. The truth is, Asian cultures traditionally have only included **fermented soy** in small amounts in their diet. Soy sauce, tempeh, natto, and miso traditionally were fermented so that the soy could be safely ingested.

Today, we are ingesting soy completely opposite of traditional wisdom in our quality & quantity. Ninety four percent of soy today is GMO (genetically modified), and if that isn't bad enough, soy is literally in EVERY SINGLE PROCESSED FOOD, either as an oil, flour, or additive. We simply eat too much of it, and bad qualities of it.

Soy is extremely high in phytic acid and trypsin inhibitors. In simpler terms, it's a pain in the rain to digest! Soy is so hard to digest, in fact, that it will also block the absorption of other minerals, vitamins, and nutrients while hangin' out in your digestive tract. In addition, soy is full of phytoestrogens, which can dangerously disrupt hormone function. Phytoestrogens mimic the hormone estrogen in our bodies. A high amount of estrogen, also known as estrogen-dominance, is the leading cause of breast cancer & infertility! What's worse, soy formula, often touted as a healthy formula alternative, has the same amount of estrogen levels as 3 birth control pills!

> *"The soybean itself is a notably inauspicious staple food; it contains a whole assortment of 'anti-nutrients' - compounds that actually block the body's absorption of vitamins and minerals, interfere with the hormonal system, and prevent the body from breaking down the proteins of the soy itself."*
>
> *-Michael Pollan*, In Defense of Food: An Eater's Manifesto

Don't be duped into thinking that soy is a good alternative for ANYTHING! Except for small amounts, preferably fermented versions like Natto, you should avoid it.

The China Study: The Whole Story

When I first read the book The China Study by Colin T. Campbell, I was initially convinced that meat & dairy would kill me. The book isn't really the full study, but rather, a conclusion from Dr. Campbell, a vegan himself. He (and other scientists) performed an observational study of 65 counties in China in the 1980s. He also performed studies on lab rats and reported those findings as well – though not technically part of the "actual" China Study.

His research is quite extensive, and to the everyday person, is a bit overwhelming. In the end, most people conclude that "this guy must know what he's talking about." He describes casein (a protein found in dairy) to be the most carcinogenic (cancer causing) substance on the planet. Whoa. That's quite a claim, Mr. Campbell. While I myself don't proclaim to be a scientist or a statistics analyst, I do love reading data, and I've noticed there are some conveniently 'cherry-picked' results in Dr. Campbell's research.

Before I begin, I must point out that Dr. Campbell serves on the advisory board to the Physicians Committee for Responsible Medicine (PCRM), a non-profit organization established in 1985 that promotes a vegan diet and higher standards for animal research. **They are an animal rights group and NOT a physician's committee,** raking in more than $6 million from the Animal Rights Foundation of Florida & $1.3 million from PETA (People for Ethical Treatment of Animals).

The China Study was NOT a controlled study, but rather an **epidemiological study** (a population based study). Because of so many different variables in different populations, epidemiological studies can never determine the causation; they only can point out correlations.

The problem is, Campbell relies on **univariate correlations** in his data to find causation. **Univariate correlations are drawn when you make a conclusion based on only one variable.** That's like saying ice cream causes drowning *(because people eat more ice cream in the summer)* or that watching television causes heart attacks *(because every heart attack victim owns a television)* or that umbrellas cause rain *(because we see higher numbers of umbrellas when it is raining)*. **See the problem with univariate correlations?**

Campbell's claim – "Children [from wealthy families] who ate the highest-protein diets were the ones most likely to get liver cancer."

Campbell's mistake - he uses a univariate correlation and fails to recognize other variables. For example, the high amount of refined breads and sugars these wealthy families were eating.

Campbell's claim - "People who ate the most animal-based foods got the most chronic disease. People who ate the most plant-based foods were the healthiest and tended to avoid chronic disease."

Campbell's mistake – The data collected from the 65 counties in China **DOES NOT** show this correlation. If animal protein **TRULY IS ASSOCIATED WITH CANCER,** then we should be able to see direct data correlating that, right? But when we actually track down his data (because he did not publish the actual data in his book), we find that animal protein **DOES NOT CORRELATE with CANCER.** Let's look at Dr. Campbell's uninterpreted data found in the actual study, Diet, Life-Style and Mortality

<u>in Rural China</u>. The Tuoli people who ate the highest amount of animal protein (about 134 grams or 22 eggs per day) were **NOT** the people with the highest amount of cancer. They ranked FOURTH actually, behind Huguan people, the Cangxi people, and the Songxian people – **ALL OF WHICH ATE LESS THAN 0.5 grams per day of animal protein!** And who gets **1ˢᵗ place** as the county with the **most heart disease? The Jiexiu people who eat 0 grams of animal protein a day!**

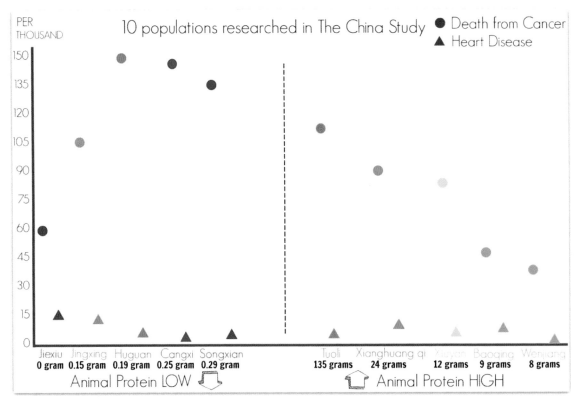

As you can see from the data, cancer is present whether animal protein consumption is high or low, with the LOWEST being from the counties who eat a moderate & balanced amount of animal protein.

> *"When we look solely at the variable "death from all cancers," the association with plant protein is +12. With animal protein, it's only +3. So why is Campbell linking animal protein to cancer, yet implying plant protein is so protective against it?"*
>
> *-Denise Minger, The China Study: Fact or Fallacy?*

Because Campbell couldn't really show that animal protein causes cancer (even in the highest animal food-eating counties—such as Tuoli, who eat 134 grams of animal protein per day), he decided to use another select variable -- cholesterol. He ignored other positive correlations to cancer in his research like higher blood glucose levels, higher consumption of refined carbs, higher consumption of vegetable oils, high alcohol intake, and stress. His own research showed schistosomiasis and hepatitis B infection as the TOP correlation with cancer, but he conveniently "cherry picked" cholesterol as a variable so he could point back at animal protein yet again.

Problem is, the link between animal food consumption and blood cholesterol levels isn't really that strong of a correlation. The Tuoli County (who ate a ton of meat) had the same cholesterol as Shanyang & Taixing County, who each consumed less than 1 gram of animal protein per day.

Dr. Campbell's claim - "Plasma cholesterol in the 90-170 milligrams per deciliter range is positively associated with most cancer mortality rates."

Did you read that correctly?

90-170 mg/dl is associated with most cancer mortality rates?! You do realize that the American Heart Association advertises that normal cholesterol is below 200 mg/dl, right? Vegans who are giving each other awards because they got their cholesterol as low as 140 mg/dl still could die of cancer?! Let me rephrase for Dr. Campbell…

"We tested 65 populations in China and their levels ranged from 90-170 mg/dl. Some of them still died of cancer. So, if you have a cholesterol number, high or extremely low – pretty much any number - you could still die of cancer."

-Me, correctly interpreting the data.

Dr. Campbell wanted to show that animal protein causes cancer. He didn't have concrete proof, so he showed that a **WIDE RANGE of cholesterol levels can cause cancer**, and he banked on the fact that most people would see the word "cholesterol" and wet their pants. Never mind the fact that it's near impossible and very dangerous to get your cholesterol below 90 mg/dl. Dr. Campbell does not mention that in **HIS OWN DATA**, wheat has a +67 correlation with heart attacks. This means there was a 67% increase in risk when wheat is consumed.

The fact is that there are MANY, MANY variables that can cause cancer, and it is wrong for Dr. Campbell to choose animal protein as the culprit. Other variables that correlate positively with cancer are high consumption of beer & liquor, high refined sugar & starch consumption, high hydrogenated fat consumption, tobacco consumption, and environmental factors.

A look at the Jiexiu County in China, a people who eat 0 grams of animal protein.

The people living in Jiexiu County in Shanxi Province eat primarily wheat flour as their staple food. They regularly eat "mianshi," a dish made of wheat flour and vegetables. A plant-based diet, no doubt, though not by their choice or beliefs. The people living in the Jiexiu County are extremely sick & poverty-stricken. The land in Jiexiu County simply won't sustain animals. The winters are cold and dry (21°F), and the summers are full of dust storms and heat waves. The people are isolated, and they are too far from the sea to obtain seafood. A study performed in 1994 showed that 90% of the females in the Jiexiu County had extremely low bone density. The Jiexiu County had the highest amount of heart attacks as well, a piece of data Dr. Campbell fails to highlight. Even more shocking, the rate of birth defects in this region is 13-15% of all births, in contrast to America's 3-4%!!

Campbell's advice – "My recommendation is that you try to avoid all animal-based products."

Dr. Campbell works very hard to convince you that animal protein is the culprit in every disease known to man, but the problem is, The China Study data does not back this up. Dr. Campbell's research on rats reports the same sketchy results…

YOU DIRTY RAT

From his experiments on rats, Dr. Campbell started by initiating cancer in the rats with high doses of aflatoxin (AF) or the virus Hepatitis B. He then fed rats a diet of either 5% animal protein or 20% animal protein. He reports that the rats (who already had cancer) who were fed a diet of 20% animal protein developed lesions of cancer, while the 5% group did not.

Campbell reports that while chemical carcinogens can initiate cancer, a diet of high animal protein can increase the progression of cancer. Because the protein he fed rats in ALL of his experiments was casein (a protein in milk), he frequently tells audiences to this day that "the casein protein found in dairy is the most carcinogenic substance on the planet."

And guess what? I agree with him. The casein Dr. Campbell used came from milk that was factory farmed, pasteurized, highly processed, and molecularly indistinguishable from real casein you'd find in raw, organic, grass-fed milk. Casein is an extremely fragile protein. Heat from pasteurization and pressure from homogenization completely destroys it, and after all that processing, it cannot bind with enzymes to be digested. It truly becomes a foreign substance in the body.

Campbell's claim – "Nutrients from animal-based foods increased tumor development while nutrients from plant-based foods decreased tumor development."

Whoa, whoa, whoa. Nutrients? We went from casein, an isolated protein (and a pasteurized, destroyed one from factory farmed animals at that), to ALL NUTRIENTS? Where's the research to back this? What about whey – the other protein in milk – and its proven anti-cancerous properties? What about all the other nutrients in animal foods, such as fat-soluble vitamins A, D, E, & K2 as well as essential fatty acids, B vitamins, Iron, Riboflavin, Calcium, Iron, Zinc, etc?

It is clear that Dr. Campbell has an agenda. Multiple critics have concluded that the book, The China Study, is simply a book advocating a vegan diet.

> "[The China Study] is basically a book-length argument for a personal opinion masquerading as hard science. The advocacy implicit in The China Study is further underscored when Campbell writes, **'Almost every time we searched for a way, or mechanism, by which protein works to produce its effects [on cancer progression], we found one!'** That, my friends, is almost the dictionary definition of confirmation bias summed up in one sentence."
>
> -Dr. Michael Eades, Advocacy, Not Science

There are many, many more flaws in Dr. Campbell's research, and while I don't mind that he personally chooses to eat a vegan diet, **his proclamation that animal products are carcinogenic (cancer-causing) is misleading and harmful to those who are looking for nutrition information to heal disease and lose weight.**

Vegan & Plant-based Diets: Don't fall for the FAD

I believe in eating a balance of all foods. I love fruits, vegetables, and grains, but I don't believe that eating them alone provides optimal nutrition. The bottom line is that plant-based diets are a modern interpretation of a healthy diet. There are no known traditional societies that have successfully thrived on a strict vegan diet. When I say "successfully," I mean those who were able to produce healthy babies and thrive for generations. Lacto-ovo-vegetarianism (a practice of including milk, eggs, and seafood but abstaining from meat) was first introduced in ancient Greece & India in the late 5th Century. After the Christianization of the Roman Empire, vegetarianism disappeared from Europe and other continents except for India. Several groups of monks abstained from meat but continued to eat fish. Vegetarianism rose again in England in the 19th century and then in America in the 20th century. John Harvey Kellogg, an early promoter of vegetarianism, proclaimed that eating animal protein led to "harmful results" such as increased libido. Morality, he claimed, was in crisis and so he created a corn flake breakfast cereal so he could save the world from the carnal nature of animal foods. The term vegan (those who abstain from all animal foods including eggs, dairy, & honey) was coined in 1944, and the American Vegan Society was founded in 1960.

Are we pretentious enough to believe that we know better than what our ancestors have known for centuries?

When Dr. Weston A. Price traveled the world in search of healthy, vibrant groups immune to disease, **he found that each healthy society DID NOT restrict animal foods.** Dr. Price was very interested in vegetarian ideas, as word of this diet was just starting to circulate in the labs of doctors & scientists.

While on Vitu Levu, a large island in the Pacific Ocean, he wrote,

"I had hoped to find on it a district far enough from the sea to make it necessary for the natives to have lived entirely on land foods. This was a matter of keen interest, and at the same time disappointment since one of the purposes of the expedition to the South Seas was to find, if possible, plants or fruits which together, without the use of animal products, were capable of providing all of the requirements for growth and for maintenance of good health and a high state of physical efficiency. I have not found a single group of primitive racial stock which was building and maintaining excellent bodies by living entirely on plant foods. I have found in many parts of the world's most devout representatives of modern ethical systems advocating the restriction of foods to the vegetable products. In every instance where the groups involved had been long under this teaching, I found evidence of degeneration."

NOT ONE of the 14 cultures Dr. Weston A. Price discovered ate diets that were vegan in nature.

Depending on where they lived and what was available to them, each of the 14 cultures ate a variety and balance of all foods including:

• Meat, primarily grass-fed - using all parts of the animals including organs and using bones to make healing broths.
• Grains, Legumes, & Seeds - typically prepared properly, soaking for 24 hours, sprouting, or using natural yeast like sourdough to break down the gluten, phytic acid, and anti-nutrients.
• Seafood - and plenty of it.

• Dairy, grass-fed - rich, high amounts of raw milk, butter, and cheese.
• Fruits & Vegetables - but only in season. They couldn't grow year-round. No green smoothies or 5-a day. Just plentiful amounts in each season they could grow it.

I wonder if we found ourselves back in nature, living off the land, where there are no grocery stores, where packaged food and supplements weren't available, and we couldn't grow fruits & vegetables year-round, if we would realize that we couldn't sustain our lives on a plant-based diet. We would probably realize that what we thought was a natural diet of only plant foods is really an unbalanced modern interpretation of a healthy diet. We'd soon realize that without the convenience of the produce department at the grocery store, we wouldn't be able to grow enough plants to sustain our lives. We would probably realize that ALL foods -- **fruits & vegetables, nuts, grains, eggs, dairy, and even meat** -- have their place in our human diet. And we'd probably realize that with each sacrifice -- whether it comes from a plant or an animal -- is for the sustainability of our lives.

A Word about Vegetarians

It should be noted that vegetarians who include dairy, eggs, and seafood in their diet (also called lacto-ovo-vegetarians or pescetarians) CAN achieve a substantially nutrient-dense diet over vegans & strict plant-based dieters. The inclusion of dairy, eggs, and seafood supplies the body with the much needed fat-soluble vitamins and important saturated fat and cholesterol needed for a healthy brain, mineral absorption, and many other functions. A carefully planned vegetarian diet can escape some of the common vegan health problems. A common problem with the avoidance of animal meat & fats, however, is the replacement of those healthy EPA & DHA stable animal fats with rancid, highly unstable vegetable & seed oils. Primarily omega-6, these vegetable & seed fats are only produced with machines and promote an inflammatory response in the body. Vegetarians, if they can focus on avoiding polyunsaturated fats, can avoid the deficiencies of EPA & DHA, common in those who eat plant-based diets.

As much as I believe in everybody choosing a diet that is right for them, I also believe in providing correct information to those who are searching. I wish I had had this information when I was eating a strict plant-based diet. I hope it helps those researching vegan diets come to a good conclusion.

"Traditional cultures are not vegan cultures. Weston Price traveled all over the world and his greatest disappointment was that he did not find a vegan culture, a group that did not use animal products. These societies extended a considerable amount of effort to get the animal products, and if they didn't hunt, and if they didn't have herds then they

ate insects, and lots of insects. So these supposedly vegetarian groups were not vegetarian, they were eating insects. The human body needs the nutrients in animal foods so desperately that it stores them. Vitamin B12 can be stored; you can have up to a ten or twelve year supply of B12. It stores vitamin A in the liver and it stores calcium and magnesium (which are more easily obtainable from animal products) in the bones. So your body can store these, and some people can go a long, long time on a vegan diet and do fine. Where you really see the problems is in the next generation. I will tell you the experience of Joe Connelly who was a dentist, who treated the people from the Self-Realization Fellowship in Los Angeles. These mothers were vegans and he saw one Down's Syndrome child after another, far, far more than you would expect in a general sampling of the population. When you try to go back to the Garden of Eden diet, when you are in a physical body, just be aware that you may end up in the living hell of nutritional deficiencies. If you go too long, for example without B12, some of these problems are irreversible."

- Sally A. Fallon

Are we being KIND by killing animals?

I believe that animals (through their meat, fats, organs, milk, and bones via broth & gelatin) can provide many nutrients that plants cannot but, more importantly, I believe that in order for meat to be truly healthy, it must be raised in a natural habitat, eating its natural diet. In my opinion, grazing animals should be allowed to, well...graze. There is a huge difference between the quality of nutrients in grass-fed, pastured beef & CAFO (Concentrated Animal Feeding Operation) beef. The same goes for pastured eggs & CAFO eggs. Not only do the Omega 3 fatty acids rise considerably when an animal is raised in a natural environment, harmful bacteria is greatly diminished. And above all, I think everyone can agree that it's much kinder for an animal to be raised outside in the fresh air rather than inside with thousands of other animals.

This is why we choose to raise our own meat. I figured (after a period of vegetarianism) that if I was going to eat meat, I'd better learn how to raise and butcher it myself. I didn't like the idea of being so disconnected from my food, and I knew that even if it would be difficult at first, I would have to connect with nature.

I wonder if the reason why some people view MEAT as MURDER is really a result of becoming disconnected from our food. Let's face it, in this modern world it's pretty rare to come across somebody who's butchered their own meat. Oh sure, we've heard of it, we know it happens somewhere far away -- but the thought of doing it ourselves?

Does being kind mean we don't eat anything living? Does being kind mean we need to sacrifice ourselves so that all can live? I've often wondered why there has never been a successful traditional society that has practiced veganism. In fact, when Weston A. Price traveled the world in search of traditional diets, he searched far and wide for vegans but only found cannibals. (http://www.westonaprice.org/blogs/cmasterjohn/2011/05/12/weston-price-looked-for-vegans-but-found-only-cannibals/) Not carnivores, cannibals. Yikes.

I believe our ancestors had more wisdom than we give them credit for. I believe their connection to the earth helped them find a balance in their diets. Partaking in all things and giving thanks for the circle of life of which we are a part. So we eat meat and show kindness in the way we respect and raise an animal. When we take that life, we do so sparingly and with gratitude like many others now and before us.

Chapter 5: TRUE Principles in REAL FOOD Weight Loss

Y ou may feel overwhelmed thinking of ALL you have to accomplish to become healthy. Stop feeling overwhelmed. You can do anything!

ANYTHING, I TELL YOU!

But you can't do it all in 2 weeks. Change takes time. I understand that this is probably the hardest thing to hear. You want to lose weight and you want to lose it now, dang it! But understand that it took some years to get that weight on, and it's not coming off instantly. In fact, you don't want it to come off fast. The faster you lose weight, the faster and easier you'll gain it back. A slow, steady weight loss, say around 1-2lbs a week, is the ideal. Please, please, please, please, don't be FOOLED by the "lose 15 pounds in 2 weeks" diets! It takes time to learn the ropes, and it takes patience. It won't be long before you start seeing results, but if you are worried about the time it will take, don't worry. The time will pass anyway. You might as well start learning and growing now.

HOW LONG WILL IT BE UNTIL YOU SEE RESULTS?

In my personal experience and from the experience of family & friends who have switched to a real food diet, weight loss should happen fairly quickly once processed foods are eliminated. If you've been eating processed foods like breakfast cereal, granola bars, crackers, cookies, etc. regularly, then your body has become accustomed to storing fake food. Toxins found in processed foods really contribute to weight gain. Once these are banned from your tummy, you'll really notice a difference. It took me about 7-8 months to lose 35 lbs.

It must be understood, however, that our bodies are all slightly different, depending on our current weaknesses and strengths. Along with having some weight to lose, most people struggle with another illness, high amounts of stress, a slow metabolism, or all three. As you switch to real food, understand that there's more to losing weight than just obsessing about what you eat. In the following section, TRUE WEIGHT LOSS PRINCIPLES, I show how changing other habits besides your diet will help promote that natural weight loss you desire. We are a society of extremes. Too often, we look for a magic pill to find the solution to our problem. In my experience, the answer is SO much simpler than we could ever imagine!

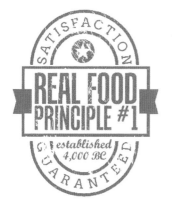

PROCESSED FOODS ARE FAKE FOODS

Every time you eat a processed, packaged food that your body doesn't recognize, you cheat yourself out of nutrition and ultimately, health. Processed & packaged foods often "seem" healthy because of claims written on the package. Phrases like "Heart Healthy," "Omega-3's," or "Fat-free" are often the hook that reels us into these purchases. Unfortunately, these foods are full of the very things that make our bodies sick & fat. About 90% of packaged/processed foods contain things like high fructose corn syrup, hydrogenated oils, artificial food colorings, artificial food flavorings, chemical stabilizers, additives, and genetically modified corn, beet sugar, and soy.

"If you're concerned about your health, you should probably avoid products that make health claims. Why? Because a health claim on a food product is a strong indication it's not really food, and food is what you want to eat"

-Michael Pollan, In Defense of Food

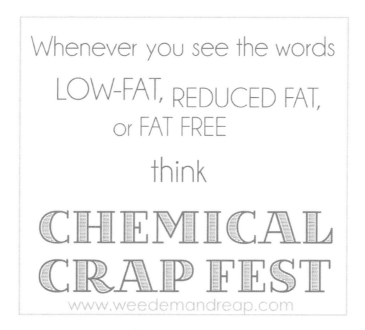

If you've done any light reading on the dangers of genetically modified foods, you'll probably recognize the name of the company behind the development of genetically modified organisms (GMOs). The company Monsanto is the evil force behind GMOs. In 2012, Monsanto made 13.5 BILLION dollars. You can literally spend hours reading about the corruption surrounding the company Monsanto – from their production of Agent Orange, which killed/deformed 1 million victims in the Vietnam War, to the successful passing of the Monsanto Protection Act signed by President Obama and hidden from the public eye. It essentially bans federal courts from halting the sale or planting of genetically modified seeds no matter what health issues may arise concerning GMOs in the future. Monsanto is infamous for their production of glyphosate (Roundup, a popular herbicide), rBGH (bovine growth hormone that was eventually outlawed), DDT (a toxic insecticide that was also eventually outlawed), and of course, Genetically Engineered Seeds. Today, Michael R. Taylor, a former Monsanto Vice President, is now the current Senior Advisor to the Commissioner of the US Food and Drug Administration. If that's not corruption, I don't know what is.

Genetically Modified Foods (GMOs): In a Nutshell

Once upon a time, farmers were conflicted. They wanted to grow and sell more food, but they didn't want to pull all the weeds in their massive fields. Luckily, a traveling salesman (known as Monsanto) swept through the town and sold a magical elixir known as an herbicide. Farmers everywhere rejoiced and their profits soared. The peasants didn't like their new poisoned food but continued to purchase from the farmers. With each application of the herbicide, farmers were unhappy to see their crops die with the weeds. They complained to Monsanto and demanded a better product. In a castle far away, on a dark and dreary night, Monsanto scientists successfully genetically modified a plant cell. Using DNA from different viruses, bacteria, plants, and animals, they successfully made Frankenfood. "It's alive!" the scientists shrieked as lightning flashed in the background. Monsanto had successfully produced a plant that could withstand the killing power of their herbicide, Roundup. Ten years and many field trials later, Monsanto was allowed by the FDA to sell their millions of seed babies to farmers & food companies. Monsanto was given all the gold in the land, as their seed babies grow and expanded to the neighboring kingdoms. Farmers skipped through the fields, joyously spraying Roundup throughout their fields. No weed pulling & no crops dying! All the problems in the world were solved! Sadly, because of the high pesticide levels in their frankenfood, plague swept throughout all the land. People got very sick, and many died. New scientists performed studies on the Frankenfood and found that animals that ate it became sick just like the people and some died from ruptured internal organs. Nobody lived happily ever after, after Monsanto came to town.

"The sheer novelty and glamor of the Western diet, with its seventeen thousand new food products every year and the marketing power - thirty-two billion dollars a year - used to sell us those products, has overwhelmed the force of tradition and left us where we now find ourselves: relying on science and journalism and government and marketing to help us decide what to eat."

-Michael Pollan,, <u>In Defense of Food</u>

The current genetically modified foods in our food supply are soy, sugar beets, corn, canola, cotton, papaya, zucchini, yellow squash, and alfalfa. Don't think you eat much of these foods?

"You may not think you eat a lot of corn and soybeans, but you do: 75 percent of the vegetable oils in your diet come from soy (representing 20 percent of your daily calories) and more than half of the sweeteners you consume come from corn (representing around 10 percent of daily calories)."

-**Michael Pollan**, In Defense of Food

So, how do we avoid frankenfood?

The safest way to avoid GMOs is to buy organic food, but before you get all upset at the thought of buying everything organic, let's make it clear that the principle is just to eat REAL food and not FAKE food. If you eat a diet high in processed foods, then yes, eating a diet high in organic processed foods is going to get expensive very fast. But eating high quality meat, seafood, dairy, grains, fruits, and vegetables isn't as much of a money strain as some would think. Buying local and in bulk are going to be your best assets when it comes to finding real food. Also, starting a vegetable garden is budget-friendly. It's time to get back in touch with real food!

ARE ANY PACKAGED FOODS OKAY?

Absolutely! Real food doesn't mean you make every single thing from scratch, but it does mean that you'll buy a lot less processed foods. Some packaged foods I still purchase are BPA-free organic coconut milk (not for drinking, it's a good replacer for sweetened condensed milk), BPA-free wild-caught salmon & tuna, jarred organic pasta sauces, salsa, sundried tomatoes, artichoke hearts, and olives, whole-grain pasta or better yet sprouted grain pasta, and organic corn tortilla chips. When purchasing packaged foods, look for organic ingredients; 5 or fewer ingredients is best.

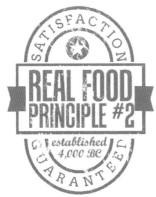

SALADS ARE NOT YOUR STAPLE

If I had a nickel for every time somebody said I probably eat tofu & salads all day to maintain my figure, I'd be a freaking millionaire. If they were to come to my house, those people would probably be shocked to see I'm eating BBQ ribs, creamy, buttery mashed potatoes, and steamed veggies, and savoring real homemade chocolate ice cream for dessert.

We need to get away from the idea that salads are the ONLY healthy food. Salads are often pushed in many diets, but the facts are that salads have large volumes and low calories – a combo that tells your body you are full, but in the end isn't very nutrient-dense.

Don't get me wrong, I love salads! In fact, I don't think there's one fruit or vegetable I don't like. But here's the problem with salads: Most people think that salads are the only healthy food. When those people want to lose weight, they start eating more salad. They get tired of salad and in the end, they give up on eating healthy. Don't give up! Fruit & vegetables are PART of a healthy diet, but not the WHOLE thing!

If we were to listen to our bodies' natural biofeedback, we wouldn't be craving salads as much as the diet world pushes. Our natural instincts would be to eat salad when we have a surplus of greens from our garden and/or during the hot summer months, when we crave 'cooling' foods. Other times, our bodies would crave 'warming' foods such as soups, meat, and comfort foods. Listen to your body. Instead of choking down salad every day for lunch, eat what you are craving – just make sure it's balanced and based on REAL FOOD.

Bottom line: Salads are wonderful, but don't make it your "go to" healthy meal.

EAT SEASONALLY & LOCALLY AND THRIVE!

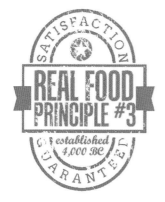

On a Sunday evening walk, my husband and I discovered that our neighbor a few houses down kept bees and sold raw honey. He was also a retired horticulturist and sold organic produce!

We also found some other neighbors who always have way too many oranges and lemons and were glad for us to take them off their hands.

Local food has been shown to have significantly higher amounts of nutrients. When you buy produce at the grocery store, you really never know how long it's been sitting and how many chemicals were used to get it to ripen. We've become so disconnected from our food, and it's time we get back in touch! Not only can you find local, healthy sources of food, you'll also learn a lot from your fellow community members. The knowledge I've acquired from all my "new" friends is priceless! We can get back to those times and use our community to help us eat healthier; we just need to search a little bit.

- Craigslist it. (www.craigslist.org) Go to your city and search 'organic', 'free-range', or 'pastured'. You'll be amazed at the results.
- Hit up Local Harvest. (www.LocalHarvest.org) It's the BEST search engine for local farms and producers.
- Cruise Facebook. I found a local group of chicken farmers that buy organic feed in bulk and save $$$ (https://www.facebook.com/BackyardChickenFarmersUnite).
- Find a local chapter of the WAPF (Weston A. Price Foundation), a group dedicated to traditional foods. They often share group deals and split on things like beef or coconut oil, saving you big $$$.
- Get to know your actual neighbors. I know this is the hardest. I mean, we see them enough, with the awkward waves when we walk out to get our mail, right? But we can do better! Build relationships and you might find healthy connections are right next door!
- Find a Farmer's Market. Search and see if your city/town has a farmer's market. This is a great way to find organic produce, and it's a really fun family activity!

FATS ARE YOUR BEST FRIEND

By now you should know that we've been pretty much scammed in the fat department.

With the invention of Crisco & margarine came the rise of heart disease & cancer and other degenerative diseases like Parkinson's, Multiple Sclerosis, and Alzheimer's. Obesity was rare before the industrialization of food, hinting that maybe, just maybe, FAT isn't making us FAT at all.

By now you should also know that YOUR ancestors have eaten lots of fat – yes even saturated fat - and have escaped these maladies. Butter & lard were the fats of choice. They were easy to produce in the home & delicious to eat! YOUR ancestors were also drinking whole milk, a complete food with a perfect amount of fat, protein, and carbohydrates. Whole, raw milk is yet ANOTHER fat-filled item that has been completely run over by the dairy industry. Is it any coincidence that when society moved away from whole milk products to highly processed dairy we became sick and fat?

Now let's talk about Low-Fat Milk, also known as 2%, 1%, or Skim. What was the reason for doing this to our beloved milk? I know what you're thinking: FAT. Too much fat. We're all fat and we want to be less fat, so the solution is to eat less fat, right?

So, what process does milk undergo to remove fat? Michael Pollan explains it well in his book, In Defense of Food.

> "To make dairy products low fat, it's not enough to remove the fat. You then have to go to great lengths to preserve the body or creamy texture by working in all kinds of food additives. In the case of low-fat or skim milk, that usually means adding powdered milk. But powdered milk contains oxidized cholesterol, which scientists believe is much worse for your arteries than ordinary cholesterol, so food makers sometimes compensate by adding antioxidants, further complicating what had been a simple one-ingredient whole food. Also, removing the fat makes it that much harder for your body to absorb the fat-soluble vitamins that are one of the reasons to drink milk in the first place."
>
> -Michael Pollan, In Defense of Food.

Processed milk, especially **LOW-FAT** milk, isn't doing you any favors. You're drinking milk that isn't nutrient-dense, and geez, isn't that why we drink it in the first place? To give our body nutrients?

Fats can be very confusing. Every bottle of oil seems to advertise its health benefits and sometimes it's just easier to grab some vegetable oil instead of researching it. I'm going to make it really easy for you. Do you want to know if a fat/oil is good for you? Simple. Just ask yourself one question:

Could I make this at home or could this only be made in a factory?

Fats that come from a factory confuse us because vegetables & seeds seem like the healthier choice, right? Naturally, we assume that the fats derived from them are healthy too.

We learned earlier that cottonseed oil (aka Crisco) is a highly processed oil, and now I'm going to give you the scoop on why it's so bad for your body. The problem with Cottonseed Oil, Sunflower oil, Soybean oil, Canola oil, Corn oil, Safflower oil, Peanut oil, Grapeseed oil, and Rice Bran oil is that they are simply TOO HIGH IN POLYUNSATURATED FATS.

Fats are divided into 3 main categories: **saturated fats, monounsaturated fats, and polyunsaturated fats.** Don't fall asleep on me yet! I'll make this short…

Our cells primarily use saturated & monounsaturated fats, and only use a small amount of polyunsaturated fats. Typically, we should eat these fats in the amounts that our body uses them. Therefore, when you eat fat, **you should be eating primarily saturated & monounsaturated and only eating a very small amount of polyunsaturated fat.**

Most seed & vegetable oils (except for palm oil, olive oil, and coconut oil) are too high in polyunsaturated fats. These highly unstable fats bond to proteins & sugars in our bodies and produce harmful toxic by-products. When eaten in large quantities, these fats will contribute to the oxidation and breakdown of our cells as well as contribute to the oxidation of low-density-lipoproteins (LDL) to create harmful oxidized cholesterol, which is atherogenic (meaning it clogs up them arteries!). Remember when Crisco was touted as healthy, while lard was labeled as "artery-clogging?" Yeah, bad call, American Heart Association! **We now know from the spike in heart disease after the consumption of Crisco & margarine (hydrogenated seed oils) increased that the high polyunsaturated fats were really the ones to blame, thanks to Proctor & Gamble and their Crisco invention.**

Fats made up mostly of saturated and monounsaturated fats are what your body was meant to eat! Your cells use saturated and monounsaturated fats for a number of vital functions, and no, they won't clog up your arteries.

HEALTHY FATS

- **Fats found in animal meat.** Remember, fat helps you digest your protein. So for heaven sakes, stop buying skinless chicken breasts and eat chicken the way it was intended! When we roast a chicken, we enjoy the crispy, herb-flavored skin as well. We also use the drippings to make delicious gravy. This makes your meal satisfying, but more importantly, it is a **WHOLE REAL FOOD** full of fat-soluble vitamins.

• **Fats found in animal dairy.** If you've been drinking skim since the 1980s, it's time to get with the times. Even if you "think" you don't like whole milk, trust me, you'll get over it just like I did. We drink whole milk and eat full-fat yogurt, full-fat cottage cheese, full-fat cream cheese, and full-fat regular cheeses. (I'll get to why we take it a step further and drink raw milk in the next chapter.)

• **Fats found in eggs & seafood.** As we talked about earlier in the calorie section, eggs pack a ton of nutrients in a small amount of food. Eggs provide your body with fat-soluble & vital B vitamins as well as minerals & antioxidants. You really can't go wrong with eggs! Seafood has a high amount of Omega-3s, particularly the essential fatty acids EPA & DHA. Seafood is an amazing food that helps promote proper cell function and improves insulin sensitivity.

• **Fats found in animal fats.** You guessed it, I'm talking about good 'ol fashioned **lard & tallow** along with **duck** or **goose fat.** You're probably going to be super sad when I tell you that the lard at the store isn't the GOOD, HEALTHY stuff. I hate to be the bearer of bad news, but the Lard you'll find at your local grocery store is hydrogenated, as well as coming from CAFO pigs. You won't find much Vitamin D from pigs kept indoors all day. Pigs are superheroes at absorbing Vitamin D from the sun, simply because they can't get sunburned. Their bodies can turn the sun's UV-B rays into Vitamin D faster than you can say "Su-ey Pig!" One tablespoon of lard contains 1,500 IU of Vitamin D! Now, what is tallow, you ask? Tallow is a fat rendered from suet, which is the fat from beef & mutton (sheep/lamb). This fat is a clean fat situated around the kidneys & loins. Extremely high in Vitamin D & K2, these fats are 55% saturated, 34% monounsaturated, and only 3% polyunsaturated. A perfect combo for your body and, more importantly, cell function!

• **Fats found in SELECT vegetable oils like olive oil, avocado oil, palm oil, and coconut oil.** These select vegetable fats are safe because the amount of saturated & monounsaturated fats are a lot higher than polyunsaturated fats.

There are a few oils from seeds that are okay in **moderation. Walnut oil, Flaxseed oil, Sesame, & Macadamia Nut Oil** are all okay, but in very small amounts and in no-heat recipes like salad dressings or mayo.

UNHEALTHY FATS

• **Crisco/shortening or hydrogenated lard** – You should know by now that these are the worst of the worst. Of the worst.

• **Fake butter spreads** – Things like Margarine, I Can't Believe it's Not Butter! spread, Crockett's spread, and even the famous Earth Balance are all high in polyunsaturated oils. They contribute to inflammation and disease, so please, please get rid of them.

• **Cooking sprays** – Things like Pam and other cooking sprays are filled with high PUFAs as well. Even if the label says 'olive oil' or omega 3's, it's still full of additives, chemicals, and most likely GMOs. Just don't use them. You can purchase misters that can be filled with any oil and work just as well as ol' Pam.

Vegetable oil, Canola oil, Corn oil, Peanut oil, or any blend that is labeled as "heart-healthy" or "omega-3's added" – Heart healthy yet full of PUFAs? Haha, you can't fool me, bottle of oil!

• **Packaged foods that contain Soybean oil, Cottonseed oil, Safflower oil, Sunflower oil, Rapeseed oil (which is canola)** – Okay, so this one will probably be the hardest one to avoid. Why? These oils are in about 90% of packaged & processed foods. Chips, cookies, crackers, pasta sauce, cake mixes, cereals, etc.

Ask yourself, what is natural? What have people thrived on for centuries? The answer is all foods, including some good ol' fashioned real fats!

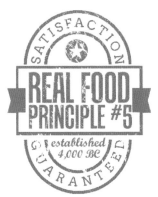

SALT & SUGAR AREN'T AS BAD AS YOU MAY THINK

Sugarcane has been used for thousands of years. Originally, people would chew the sugarcane in an effort to extract its sweetness. Planting, harvesting, and extracting the sweet juice from the sugarcane plant is pretty labor intensive. To make sugar crystals, one would have to grind the plant to extract the juice, boil down the juice to concentrate it, and then dry it in the sun to create crystallized sugar. Around the 16th century, beets were discovered to contain sucrose as well, and thus began the harvesting of beets for their sugar. It was found that beets were easier to grow because they could grow in a wider range of climates. Also, the refining process was simple and so many people began to jump on the beet wagon.

Genetically Modified sugar beets were first introduced to the world by the company Monsanto in 2008. Remember Monsanto? Luckily, cane sugar HASN'T been genetically modified yet. It's not because they haven't tried; scientists have been working on making cane sugar GMO for YEARS, but have failed due to the difficult genetic structure of cane sugar. Keep holdin' out, little sugar cane buddy! Never give up, never surrender!

Currently, there is no law that requires labeling of whether the manufacturer used beet sugar or cane sugar. It is estimated that about HALF of all sugar sold in the US is from sugar beets. This is bad because almost all sugar beets are genetically modified.

Because there is no law that requires sugar manufacturers to label whether their sugar is BEET sugar or CANE sugar, you really don't know what you're getting. It could be the non-GMO and therefore healthier cane sugar OR it could be the GMO beet sugar OR it could be a mixture of both...problem is, there's no real way of knowing unless it says 100% pure cane sugar. It's important for you to know what you're feeding your family.

Although white sugar seems to be a common ingredient in MANY recipes, it's a highly processed item and isn't great to eat regularly. If you want to lose weight, heal your body, regulate your hormones, and improve behavior in your children, then I wouldn't suggest purchasing or baking with a lot of white sugar. You don't have to COMPLETELY avoid it. I believe that a huge reason for real food failure is trying to be perfect. A rule in our house is that we don't bring the highly processed sugar into our home, but if we are at a family gathering or event and we want to partake, then we do. We know it's not the best. We avoid it. We bring food to events with REAL sugar. But we also avoid being too strict.

Choose from any of these sweeteners for your home cooking/baking:

- Local Honey
- Maple Syrup, Grade B
- Stevia
- Unrefined brown cane sugar (such as Rapadura or Sucunat)
- Coconut sugar

(If you can only find 100% cane sugar that is white, I wouldn't stress too bad about it, though I would use it sparingly. You're doing better by not eating GMO beet sugar, but it's best to depend on unrefined sugars as a sweetener.)

If you've researched health on the internet, you've probably come across many articles demonizing sugar. Many people claim that sugar is horribly addicting, feeds candida & cancer, and pretty much makes any illness worse. Satan's spawn, that sugar. They lump all sugar from high fructose corn syrup to sweet potatoes in the same category and call it all bad.

The truth is, as long as you are eating natural forms of sugar, it's very beneficial. Our cells use sugar (in the form of glucose) as the preferred source of energy. Our bodies are supplied with glucose from grains, root vegetables like carrots, regular potatoes, sweet potatoes, and FRUITS. We also get glucose from sweeteners like honey, maple syrup, coconut sugar, and unrefined cane sugar. What happens when you go on a complete NO-sugar diet and deprive your body of these foods? At first you feel great, but it comes at a cost, and here's why:

When you deprive your body of all sugar, your body has to figure out another way to make glucose. Your body will either use fat to make sugar (Lipolysis) or protein to make sugar (Gluconeogenesis). At first, people are like, **"Yeah! Use my fat to make sugar!"**

But, depriving your body of glucose puts your body in stress mode. Your body works hard, producing adrenaline and cortisol to keep up with the demand. Adrenaline and cortisol give you energy, but the **human body is not meant to live in stress mode for extended periods of time.**

You are essentially telling your body, "Hey, I'm starving you – figure it out!" to which your body replies, "Okay, but once you start eating glucose again, I'm gonna store it up like nobody's business! I gotta pack on weight just in case you try to pull this stunt again!"

Eating a balance of all foods and sticking with health sweeteners like those listed above will be better for you in the long run. If you feel that you are sensitive to sugar or feel you are hypoglycemic, don't be so quick to demonize sugar. People often label their bodies as hypoglycemic when they really are experiencing hyponatremia (low blood salt levels) by drinking gobs of water because it's "healthy" instead of just drinking when they're thirsty.

SALT

Salt is yet another food that has been vilified by the "health community." Salt, they say, contributes to high blood pressure & weight gain. A low salt intake is recommended for everyone (especially those with high blood pressure).

The American Heart Association & the American Diabetes Association both want you to eat less sodium. So, what's the truth? Should we be watching that salt intake?

I say NO & here are a couple reasons why:

1. A study in 2003 showed that a reduction in salt intake only lowered systolic blood pressure by 4 points & diastolic by only 1 point.
2. That same study also showed that a reduction in salt intake increased triglyceride levels, LDL levels, and stress hormones.
3. Salt supports hydration, especially when we experience fluid loss due to exercise.
4. Salt is a de-stressor and helps clear the stress hormone Cortisol from the blood.

Well, why in the heck does everyone have an issue with salt nowadays? It's because when people crave salt, they tend to eat fast food French fries or packaged potato chips (both cooked in bad oils). Those hydrogenated poly-unsaturated oils are wreaking havoc on your health, but instead we place the blame on salt.

Your body works hard to maintain the perfect amount of sodium in your blood. If you disrupt that balance by either reducing your salt intake or drinking too much water when your body isn't thirsty, you'll suffer the consequences in the form of low blood pressure, fatigue, cold hands & feet, low metabolism, and higher stress hormones.

The solution is simple: Eat a good quality salt, particularly a sea salt that is gray, red, brown, black, or even pink in color, indicating high amounts of trace minerals. White salt means it's been bleached and doesn't contain a lot of minerals. And how much should you eat? Well, it's even simpler: Trust in your body. Salt your food until it tastes perfect **to you.** Your body knows how much salt it needs. If something tastes too salty, it probably is. If something tastes like it needs more salt, by all means, use it!

HEAL YOUR GUT, HEAL YOUR BODY

Food allergies and sensitivities are becoming an epidemic. It is estimated that 1-in-5 Americans now have some sort of food allergy. A study in the Journal of Allergy and Clinical Immunology found that ER visits at the Boston Children's Hospital for allergic reactions more than doubled from 2001 to 2006! What could be causing all these reactions? Well, there are many theories – GMOs, too much of a hygienic environment, and a delayed introduction of foods - but everybody is in agreement on one thing: Up till about 50 years ago, allergies were rare, and now they are rampant.

Have you ever wondered how your body became allergic or sensitive to a food in the first place? To understand how this happened, you must first understand **dysbiosis**, or what is also referred to as **"the leaky gut syndrome."** To put it simply, at some time, your body's intestinal flora and wall became compromised. Stress, illness, a sterile environment, prescription medication, anti-biotics, and genetically modified foods all reduce the good bacteria and break down the wall in your intestinal tract. Essentially you've developed a "leaky gut."

A leaky gut is no bueno. Why? Because our food was not meant to be absorbed into our bloodstream until it has been broken down into the correct nutrients. If a food particle - like, for example, from that sandwich you ate - gets absorbed into your bloodstream at the wrong time, all hell breaks loose. Basically what happens is your body cannot recognize that food particle, it is viewed like a foreign substance, and your immune system has tagged it as "BAD." Next time you eat that food, your body raises up the red flag and attacks.

Did you know that Nexium & Prevacid were the top 2nd & 3rd medications prescribed in 2012? Yikes. Lots o' people got their stomachs in knots. It's time to get off the drugs and heal that gut!

There is a mistaken belief in modern medicine that if a person is allergic or sensitive to a food, then that person must avoid that food until they are no longer allergic. The sad thing is, **simply avoiding that food will not magically make the body heal.** There are many actions that you must take to promote healing in your gut.

Inside our intestines are little organisms, often called "good bacteria," that help us digest and absorb our food. We want this good bacteria, we NEED it. Many things can cause our intestinal flora to become out-of-balance. Stress, illness, a sterile environment, prescription medication, anti-biotics, and even eating a Standard American Diet (SAD) including genetically modified foods (GMOs) can reduce the number of healthy gut bacteria.

Some symptoms of poor gut flora are:
• Gluten Intolerance
• IBS, Crohn's
• Gas
• Bloating
• Cramps
• Indigestion
• Headaches
• Food Allergies
• Seasonal Allergies
• Frequent Colds & Flus
• Joint Pain & Stiffness

Benefits to having a balanced gut flora:
• Resolution of digestive symptoms.
• Helps digest sugars, proteins, minerals, & fats. Resolves digestive issues, aka bloating, gas, diarrhea, constipation.
• Strengthens the intestinal lining to help block out pathogens, allergens, & toxins.
• Strengthens the immune system.
• Aids against the overgrowth of certain microorganisms, like yeast (candida).
• Produces specific vitamins.

"In the normal scheme of things, we'd never have to think twice about replenishing the bacteria that allow us to digest food. But since we're living with antibiotic drugs and chlorinated water and antibacterial soap and all these factors in our contemporary lives that I'd group together as a 'war on bacteria,' if we fail to replenish [good bacteria], we won't effectively get nutrients out of the food we're eating."

– Sandor Katz

HOMEMADE FERMENTED FOODS ARE THE KEY:

Our ancestors were smarty pants. They knew fermented foods were the key to a healthy gut and therefore a healthy body. Fermented beverages and fermented foods have been dated as far back as 4,000 BC. The fermentation process kept food for longer times, allowing cultures to sustain themselves through the winter. Bread, cheese, pickles, yogurt – these were all fermented properly before the industrialization of food. When we stopped canning in the home and started purchasing canned goods from the store, we lost the art of lacto-fermentation. Our ancestors had jars of sauerkraut & lacto-fermented cucumber pickles stored in the cellar. Today, the store bought versions do not carry beneficial bacteria in the amounts like they used to. Today (and especially in America due to lack of culture-specific foods), we just don't have enough beneficial bacteria in our guts.

You've probably heard of probiotics before and have chuckled at the familiar Jamie Lee Curtis commercials promoting Activia (a brand of yogurt) to ensure a regular bowel movement every day. Well, Miss Jaime Lee Curtis is both right and wrong. While yogurt helps to improve your digestion, store bought versions are not optimal. Your body needs two things...**PREBIOTICS & PROBIOTICS.** Without these foods, your body cannot perform efficient digestion. And we all want efficient digestion, am I right?

Probiotics help colonize your gut with essential bacteria. Prebiotics help feed that good bacteria. Together, they help you have a superhero system.

Good Sources of Probiotics
• Natural Yeast/Sourdough Bread
• Raw aged cheese
• Yogurt
• Kombucha
• Water Kefir
• Fermented & Cultured Vegetables
• Fermented Condiments
• Probiotic Supplements (only BioKult brand)

Good Sources of Prebiotics
• Jicama
• Chicory
• Endive & Dandelion greens
• Artichoke
• Onions
• Asparagus
• Garlic

"The proliferation of lactobacilli in fermented vegetables enhances their digestibility and increases vitamin levels. These beneficial organisms produce numerous helpful enzymes as well as anti-biotic and anti-carcinogenic substances. Their main by-product, lactic acid, not only keeps vegetables and fruits in a state of perfect preservation, but also promotes the growth of healthy flora throughout the intestine."

-Sally A. Fallon

SEAL YOUR GUT

Along with including homemade probiotic and prebiotic foods in your diet, it's equally important to include grass-fed gelatin as well. Gelatin heals & seals the mucosal lining of the intestinal tract and aids in the assimilation of nutrients. Gelatin is the same collagen that is found in our bones, skin, and cartilage. Gelatin is an easily digestible protein and works as an anti-inflammatory as well. **Gelatin is VITAL** to heal a damaged gut.

You can obtain gelatin from homemade bone broth, the drippings from whole meats (often used to make gravy), or in a powdered supplement form. Be sure to get the best powdered brand, made from grass-fed animals. I purchase Great Lakes Gelatin online. I use the beef unflavored gelatin for use in puddings & desserts, and I also use the hydrolysate formula (doesn't congeal in liquid) to take as a daily supplement.

What to do if your food allergies/sensitivities don't heal

Some people have small sensitivities while others have major allergies. For severe allergies or neurological problems like Autism, it may do you well to look into the healing GAPS diet. The GAPS diet was created by Dr. Natasha Campbell-McBride, a neurologist who healed her son's Autism by healing his leaky gut syndrome. You can find her book & intro guide online at www.gapsdiet.com.

For skin issues, including eczema & psoriasis, you can read more about my friend Emily's amazing protocol that healed her daughter's extreme eczema. It is similar to a real food diet, along with some specific protocol for eczema sufferers. Here's the link: http://holisticsquid.com/the-eczema-cure/

If you're on the fence and trying to decide whether you should jump on the GAPS diet or simply incorporate more probiotics/prebiotics/gelatin into your diet, check out my friend Cara's article at http://www.healthhomehappy.com/2013/03/i-dont-need-gaps-die.html for more clarification. She's the expert!

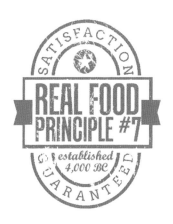

DON'T UNDERESTIMATE THE POWER OF
SLEEP

I would bet that every single one of you is underestimating the power of sleep! Did you know that **our bodies can withstand years of poor nutrition, but if we go more than 11 days without sleep, our bodies WILL DIE?** It's true. People who have tried to set a world record for longer than 11 days have actually died! Sleep deprivation is so damaging to the body that it is used in war as a form of torture! Isn't it amazing that we spend so much time analyzing our diets, yet we forget about the quality and quantity of our sleep? Are you torturing your body during the night but expecting it to perform miracles during the day?

"Health is a net result of ALL of our thoughts, emotions, social interactions, sleep quantity and quality, hydration levels, and a lot more than just whether the cow you're eating ate grass or corn. In the grand scheme of things, all that dietary small stuff that the healthosphere seems obsessed with is minutiae. Absolutely minutiae. Eating grass-fed beef to be healthy is like fighting a forest fire with an eye dropper if you aren't sleeping well, hate your life, spend most of your time doing mundane and uninspiring work, are financially stressed, never go outdoors, skip meals, and eat an inadequate amount of calories."

-Matt Stone, <u>Diet Recovery 2</u>

How much sleep should you be getting? Experts agree that 8-9 hours of sleep is optimal, and the "early to bed, early to rise" rule is especially important.

TIPS FOR THOSE WHO HAVE TROUBLE SLEEPING

Wanting to get a good night's rest but not being able to sleep is a frustrating place to be! Many factors can play into why you are not sleeping well, so let's go over some tips to help you out.

- **Supplement temporarily with Melatonin.** Melatonin is the body's natural sleep hormone. When it gets dark outside, our pineal gland is stimulated and melatonin is released into the bloodstream. Because of the invention of electricity, we naturally stay up later than our ancestors did, and our bodies often don't produce enough Melatonin before bedtime. It is recommended that you take your dose at about 8pm, which should get you tired by 10pm.

• **Supplement temporarily with an Amino Acid.** Trouble sleeping could indicate that your body is producing a low amount of neurotransmitters. Neurotransmitters are made from amino acids, and amino acids are in the proteins we eat. Ideally, our bodies use amino acids from protein to make neurotransmitters. If you have been under physical, emotional, or social stress, then your body may be experiencing a neurotransmitter deficiency. Take Dr. Ross's free online survey (http://www.moodcure.com/take_the_mood_type_questionnaire.html) to see if you are deficient in any neurotransmitters. Often by balancing these out, you can notice a big change in your sleep patterns.

• **Protect your eyes from electronic screens.** "Short-wavelength blue lights," a type of light emitted by televisions, cellphones, and computer screens, have been shown to cause melatonin suppression. By using these devices after sundown, you are effectively suppressing the production of melatonin and setting yourself up for a bad night's sleep. Don't worry; there are some great solutions to this! You can install a free program, such as f.lux (http://stereopsis.com/flux/), on your computer & cellphone to help dim your screen at the start of sundown each day. It is synced with your local time-zone, so it automatically turns down the screen for you. Another solution is to purchase amber-lensed glasses. You can purchase them for about $8 on Amazon.com and just slip them on each evening. Plus, you'll look super cute wearing them.

• **Make your bedroom the optimal sleeping zone.** You'll want to focus on 3 things – a cool, dark, and quiet bedroom. Optimal temperature is 76 degrees. To make your room dark, you can either buy blackout curtains or wear a sleeping mask. Even something like a blinking phone or an alarm clock should be covered! For a quiet room, try ear plugs. You should still be able to hear your children and carry on a conversation, but all the little sounds of the house, like the ticking of a clock or the creaks in the night, can be blocked out.

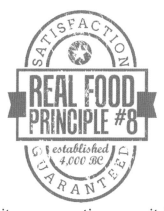

BALANCE, BALANCE, BALANCE!

The fact that I said this 3 times should tell you how important I think it is! Just in case you aren't getting it, I'll say it one more time…wait for it…

BALANCE!

Health is NOT JUST eating better or avoiding GMOs. Health is a combination of all things – diet, sleep, how you handle stress, your family relationships, and your movement!

Another thing to mention here is you are only as good as your stress level. If you are trying to eat a real food diet but are feeling restricted and never allow yourself to sample the dessert tray at your local church function, then you will cause yourself more stress and harm in not eating that poly-unsaturated fat, GMO-filled dessert than eating it in the first place! Alternatively, allowing yourself to eat that dessert, yet feeling stressed and guilty about it afterwards will also be just as bad. The solution?

JUST RELAX & EAT THE FOOD!

Trust me, worrying and stressing about food will be more harmful than actually eating the "bad" food in the first place!

"The answer is much simpler and easier, and is what most people's bodies are crying for them to do anyhow. And that is get sufficient rest, sleep, and relaxation for starters and pair that with a superabundance of nutritious foods with an emphasis on eating plentiful amounts of what I call the anti-stress S's - starch, sugar, salt, and saturated fat – and more importantly calories. Top this off by spending sufficient time doing enjoyable activities with a little supplemental, well-designed exercise."

-Matt Stone, Diet Recovery

THE 80/20 RULE

In our home, we institute the 80/20 rule. This means we eat nourishing foods 80% of the time and allow ourselves to not worry about it 20% of the time. We don't calculate exactly the precise amount; we honestly just do the best we can.

Here are some good tips for sticking to that 80/20 RULE:

• **80% of the time**, we strive to put nourishing foods in our bodies. This means we only bring nourishing foods into the home. We don't store processed or packaged foods in our pantry. We don't buy Crisco, canola, or vegetable oils. In our fridge we have organic dairy products, mostly organic fruits & vegetables, nuts & seed, and some meats/broths/animal fats like butter, lard, or tallow. In our pantry we have coconut oil, grains, some BPA-free canned goods, some home-canned goods, and spices/seasonings.
• **20% of the time**, when we eat at family or friend gatherings, we eat whatever is served, happily and with thankfulness. When we eat out, we don't ask if the oil is NON-GMO or if the vegetables are organic. We eat what sounds good to us, enjoy our meal, and then go back to our home where nourishing foods reside.

The key here is HOME. What you have at home you will eat, so take it from me, don't buy fruit snacks, chips, crackers, ice cream, frozen pizza, etc. Trust me, you will fill up your 20% rather fast from eating outside of the home, so **keep it real where you live.**

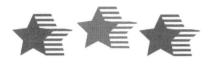 # SUPPLEMENTS: to take or not to take

Ideally, if you are eating a traditional real food diet, you shouldn't have to supplement very much at all. The fact is, this world we live in has toxins and soil depletion. If you are coming back from a SAD (Standard American Diet), then you may need some supplements to assist in the healing process.

Supplementing will NEVER trump a bad diet, so it's good to remember **not** to rely on supplementation as the primary source of nutrition.

THE SUPPLEMENT EVERYBODY SHOULD TAKE:

Fermented Cod Liver Oil:

You've probably heard of "Cod Liver Oil" but wonder why it needs to be fermented. And you're probably gagging just thinking about it. Most cod liver (& fish oil for that matter) on the market today has been extracted through heat. Heat destroys enzymes & nutrients; therefore, almost all of the fish oils/liver oils on the market today are rancid.

Fermented fish liver oils are extracted through a cold process, therefore aiding in the digestion and assimilation of their nutrients. It only takes a day to extract oil if heated, but it usually takes about 6 months if fermented. At the turn of the century, when the industrialization of food became popular, manufacturers decided to skip the 6-month fermentation step to reduce costs.

Your grandma may have taken cod liver oil as a child, but it was probably during this time when cod liver was extracted with heat and was therefore not as beneficial as your great-grandmother's fermented version.

Fermented Cod liver oil is an ancient food. It has been used for thousands of years as a sacred food to boost one's health. As far back as 200 B.C, the Romans would ferment fish liver oil and credit their strength & vitality to it. According to anthropologist William Stefansson's book, Scandinavian fishermen believed in the nearly magical powers of cod or halibut liver oil, and some would drink a wineglassful every morning. In the book Nutrition & Physical Degeneration, Dr. Weston A. Price noted that every single one of the 14 isolated traditional cultures he visited ingested FCLO regularly as a vital real food supplement to their diets.

Fermented Cod liver oil is the MOST nutrient-dense food on the planet! FCLO is rich in eicosapentaenoic acid (EPA) and docasahexaenoic acid (DHA). EPA & DHA are essential fatty acids found in Omega 3 fat. EPA & DHA are vital nutrients that maintain the health of the brain & eyes, regulate cell activity & healthy cardiovascular function, and play an extremely important role during fetal brain development! EPA & DHA have also been known to ease the symptoms associated with Alzheimer's disease, Dementia, Depression, Autism, ADHA, Aspergers, and Multiple Sclerosis. FCLO also contains extremely high amounts of Vitamins A & D. One teaspoon of FCLO contains 9500 IU of Vitamin A and 1950 IU of Vitamin D! FCLO has also been known to be a fertility boosting super food and inflammation buster! The brand of Fermented Cod Liver Oil I trust is Green Pastures. I like the cinnamon flavor the best. They also come in capsule form if you don't want to taste it. I prefer the Fermented Cod Liver Oil/Butter Oil Blend because Dr. Price found this combination provided the best results in healing. The butter oil found in the FCLO from Green Pastures comes from grass-fed cows so you know you're getting the highest quality.

Additional Supplements:

Magnesium – Many people are low in magnesium, as it's difficult to obtain magnesium from food because of the depletion of the soil. Dr. Carolyn Dean, author of <u>The Magnesium Miracle</u>, lists common symptoms associated with magnesium deficiency:

- Acid Reflux
- Adrenal Fatigue
- Anxiety
- Infertility
- Panic Attacks
- PMS
- Menstrual Cramps
- High Blood Pressure
- Diabetes
- Fibromyalgia

- Constipation
- Migraines
- Morning Sickness
- Heart Attacks
- IBS
- Inflammation
- Insomnia
- Kidney Stones
- Seizure

Magnesium is especially beneficial during pregnancy for proper fetal growth. It also helps sustain mom throughout pregnancy, and it's known for staving off morning sickness. In fact, low magnesium levels are common in pregnant mothers who experience hyperemesis gravidarum (extreme morning sickness). Gosh, I wish I would have known that with my horrible pregnancies! Magnesium is best taken as a Magnesium oil spray or ionic drops. Magnesium pills aren't absorbed as readily and can cause diarrhea. (Ask me how I know.)

Gelatin – Grass-fed gelatin is a great source of protein and is extremely healing to the gut. It also gives you great skin, hair, and nails as well as providing great support to your bones & joints! If you've got arthritis or inflammation, gelatin can help heal that connective tissue. Gelatin is more of a food source than an actual supplement, and you can make some awesome fruit snacks, puddings, and jello with it. If you don't want to cook with it, you can purchase hydrolyzed gelatin, which is gelatin that doesn't gel, so you can just mix it in with orange juice or water and chug it.

Probiotics – It's best to obtain your probiotics in a natural form like yogurt, milk kefir, water kefir, kombucha, sauerkraut, or fermented vegetables & condiments, BUT if you are experiencing some serious digestive issues and additionally need to take it in supplement form, the ONLY brand I'd trust is BioKult. All other probiotics are proprietary strains and really don't have high enough strength to be beneficial.

Essential Herbal Oils – Herbal essential oils are anti-bacterial, anti-fungal, anti-tumor, anti-parasitic, and anti-septic. They are unique in that they can cross the cellular membrane because their molecules are so small, which is pretty amazing. The fact that essential oils are 50-70 times more concentrated than the herb explains why it is so effective. I use essential oils regularly in my home. From cuts & sprains, to joint pain, mood uplifting, cleaning supplies, and DIY products, it's a staple for us.

Melatonin – This is a great temporary supplement you can use if you are having trouble sleeping or you are trying to go to bed earlier to heal your metabolism & improve your health. I'm a night owl, but I'm trying to change that. I take a dose of melatonin around 9pm so I am sure to be tired by 10pm. Works great, and I plan on discontinuing it once I "set" my sleep cycle.

Amino Acids – If you are having some mood issues, I highly suggest reading The Mood Cure, by Dr. Julia Ross. Your body uses amino acids (from proteins) to create neurotransmitters and provide stability in the brain. An imbalance of neurotransmitters could mean you need to supplement temporarily with an amino acid. Check it out!

Iodine – Since the 1970s, our iodine consumption has dropped dramatically. Additionally, fortified foods contain chemicals that inhibit our absorption of iodine. Even if we eat a balanced real food diet, we are exposed to many environmental factors that prevent our bodies from absorbing iodine. Iodine is necessary for healthy thyroid function and metabolism as well as the prevention of breast cancer. It's a very important supplement every woman should take. I also recommend reading Lynne Farrow's book, The Iodine Crisis, for more information.

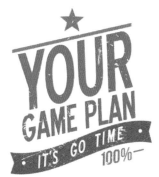

Chapter 6: Getting Started with Real Food

First and foremost, I cannot stress to you the importance of NOT stuffing your face with crap in preparation for this new dietary change. First of all, it PLANTS the IDEA in your head that you won't enjoy food at all in your new lifestyle and that you will never eat junk food again (which isn't true at all). You can still have whatever your little heart desires, in moderation, which by the way will be super easy to do after you have broken your addiction. Eat how you would normally eat before you make your real food change. Even if it is pizza and soda, that's okay as long as it's your normal. Don't think "Hmmm, what is the most delicious, unhealthy thing I can eat before my new real food change? Oreos, ice cream, and hotdogs and......" You get the point. Don't fall into this thought process. Eat primarily nutritious foods and you'll be set!

- Remember that ALL FOOD GROUPS are nourishing to your body.
- Remember that your ancestors have included ALL FOOD GROUPS for centuries.
- Remember that a traditional diet heals, and modern foods slowly kill.
- Remember you don't have to be perfect to experience awesome weight loss and amazing disease reversal.
- Remember that it takes time to accomplish a lifestyle change, and you won't be able to do it overnight.

Your NEW Real Food Rules

1. Take all the diet plans you've followed, all the healthy eating lists you've found on the internet, all the magazines you've saved, and chuck them all OUT THE WINDOW. Or better yet, burn them. We don't want to spread crappy health rules to the homeless guy.

2. Eat nourishing foods about 80% of the time – this includes homemade food made with real ingredients.

3. Chillax and "just eat the food" about 20% of the time – this includes everything that happens OUTSIDE of your home (family gatherings, going out to eat, church functions).

4. Eat when you are hungry.

5. Drink when you are thirsty.

6. Don't restrict fat, carbohydrates, protein, real salts, or real sugar.

7. Try to find the best quality of each food group.

8. Realize you are awesome.

Real Food GROUPS: The Basics

FRUITS & VEGETABLES:

Organic is best because there are way less pesticides (and no GMOs ya'll), but honestly just do the best you can. If you can't buy organic, don't sweat it, just shop the sales. Eat what you love. There is a huge variety for you to enjoy, and there's gotta be something you like! Eating seasonally will not only make fruits and vegetables cheaper, they will also be healthier. You may even want to consider starting a vegetable garden; it's actually really fun and easier than you think. Ever heard of the "dirty dozen, clean fifteen" rule? This is a great guide to use if you can't purchase all organic produce.

Dirty Dozen	Clean Fifteen
(Crazy amount of pesticides/herbicides – try to purchase only organic)	(Hardly any pesticides/herbicides – okay to buy the regular stuff)
1. apples	1. asparagus
2. celery	2. avocado
3. cherry tomatoes	3. cabbage
4. cucumber	4. cantaloupe
5. grapes	5. corn
6. hot peppers	6. eggplant
7. nectarines (imported)	7. grapefruit
8. peaches	8. kiwi
9. potatoes	9. mangoes
10. spinach	10. mushrooms
11. strawberries	11. onions
12. sweet bell peppers	12. papayas
…plus collards & kale	13. pineapples
…plus summer squash & zucchini	14. sweet peas (frozen)
	15. sweet potatoes

A WORD ABOUT GRAINS, BEANS, NUTS, & SEEDS

One of the most interesting things that Dr. Weston A. Price discovered when he visited each of the 14 traditional societies is that they ALWAYS prepared their grains properly. It was ridiculous to them to eat a nut without soaking it first, or to grind a grain into flour and bake bread without a pre-soak time. This is because these traditional societies knew that grains, beans, nuts, and seeds are full of anti-nutrients and are extremely difficult to digest unless prepared properly. This is the same reason why grains can be stored longer than any food. They just won't break down on their own. Everybody used to prepare their grains properly; in fact, your great-grandma might remember that the instructions on the oatmeal box recommended an overnight soak before cooking. Those instructions were removed with the invention of quick oats and microwavable oats.

There are 3 options to choose when preparing grains (and beans, nuts, and seeds) properly – you can **soak, sprout, or sour leaven.** You don't have to do all three, you just have to choose one, and once you get the hang of it, it'll be easy peasy lemon squeezy…

Do you have to soak, sprout, or sour leaven **EVERY SINGLE TIME?** No. Like I talked about earlier, it's important to live the 80/20 rule and avoid stress when it comes to eating. I'm giving you the education, and instead of feeling overwhelmed you're going to take this knowledge and slowly start incorporating these principles before you eat grains, beans, nuts, or seeds. Don't feel discouraged or overwhelmed with this new information.

BEANS, NUTS, & SEEDS

Beans are budget-friendly. They are a great extender to any meal. Again, organic is best, but just do the best you can. Buying organic beans isn't going to make the difference between you losing weight or not, but I like to give a shout out that organic means less pesticides and, well, that's always a good thing. The best way to cook any bean or legume is to **soak it first for 8-24 hours** on your kitchen counter covered in water with a tablespoon of an acidic medium such as **apple cider vinegar, whey, yogurt, or lemon.** (This is also in the order of my fav acidic mediums to use. Lemon's just not my fav.) Soaking with a tablespoon of an acidic medium simply helps release that phytic acid. And bonus, no more need for Beano! Gas isn't an issue in beans that have been soaked before cooking. After soaking, your cooking time will be cut in half.

Nuts & seeds can be budget-friendly as well if purchased in bulk and stored in the freezer. Before consuming, however, they offer your body optimal nutrition and easy digestion if you **soak for 8-12 hours in plain filtered water** on your kitchen counter. If I'm having yogurt with nuts or oatmeal with nuts for breakfast or using nuts as a topper on pancakes or crepes that morning, I simply start a handful of nuts soaking before I go to bed the night before. You can also soak, drain, and dehydrate nuts to store in your freezer and they'll be ready to go.

GRAINS

Grains are also budget-friendly and easy to purchase in bulk. They also store well because of all those anti-nutrients. Grains are divided into two categories -- **GLUTEN** grains and **NON-GLUTEN GRAINS.** Those who are sensitive or allergic to gluten tend to avoid those gluten grains (and also try to convince everybody of their horrible-ness), but what many gluten-free people don't realize is that if they just prepared their gluten grains properly, they may notice they aren't sensitive to gluten at all (of course those who are allergic should take care when introducing gluten grains back into their diet).

NON-GLUTEN GRAINS

Oats Although oats don't have gluten in them, they are often grown next to wheat fields. This is why gluten-intolerant people purchase gluten-free oats. If you prepare your grains properly, however, you won't have to worry about the chance of a couple of flattened wheat kernels in there.

Rice, White or Brown There are many different varieties of rice. Most diet gurus would lump white rice in with white flour and white sugar and label it as a "bad food." The truth is that brown rice carries with it extremely high amounts of phytic acid along with an unhealthy dose of poly-unsaturated fats. Traditional societies knew this and would pound up the brown rice with a mortar & pestle, then sift out the bran to make the minerals more available through the removal of the bran and subsequent phytic acid. It's also the reason why Asian cultures prefer white varieties of rice. I'm not going to say which is better – white or brown - because I think they can both be included in a healthy diet. I'll leave it up to you and how your body feels when you eat it. **When eating brown rice, just be sure to soak it well with an acidic medium for 24 hours. White doesn't need that long of a soak, only about 4-8 hours. We still eat some brown rice, but also eat white varieties such as Basmati or Jasmine.**

Quinoa Quinoa is high in protein and is often a great substitution for meat in dishes. However, its rise in popularity is quickly making it an unsustainable food. We don't eat a ton of it and save it for special dishes. I personally like the white quinoa better than the red.

Corn is tricky because so much of it is GMO today. Traditionally, corn is prepared by soaking in lime water for 2 weeks, and then it is ground up into a paste shaped into tortillas, fried into chips, or mixed with lard and made into tamales. It's probably the last grain that is being prepared correctly. Because organic corn is expensive and making homemade properly-prepared corn products is time-consuming, we buy in bulk and use it mostly to make popcorn, or we grind the corn in our grain mill to make cornmeal to be used in a soaked corn muffin recipe. We purchase organic corn tortillas and chips at our health food store when we need them, but we don't eat them very often, simply because of the expense.

Buckwheat, Amaranth, Millet, Kasha, Teff These are other non-gluten grains that are used frequently in side dishes around the world. Feel free to include them in recipes if you want.

GLUTEN GRAINS

Wheat berries are ground into wheat flour. Wheat has a bit of a history. Today's wheat is a hybrid wheat, but not to be confused with GMO. Hybrid means that a special variety was formed by combining certain characteristics in other grains. It's a natural method of producing a new variety, but it doesn't come without its drawbacks. Today's wheat has a stronger stalk, higher amounts of gluten, and more anti-nutrients. This is why many people who have an intolerance to wheat will try older heirloom varieties such as **Spelt, Emer, and Einkorn** instead. I really love the taste of Spelt, but it is not cheap. We stick with wheat and prepare it many different ways depending on the recipe. We will **soak wheat flour overnight** in recipes such as muffins, biscuits, pancakes, etc. We will also use **soaked methods** or **sour leavening methods** to bake bread. And finally, we will use already **sprouted flour** we store in our freezer for last minute baking. Of course we're not perfect and have been known to buy a loaf of crusty artisan bread from the health food store. If you can't make homemade bread, find the best brand possible. Store bought breads can have many chemicals and additives you don't want to eat on a daily basis. You'll want to look for simple ingredients you can recognize, like whole-wheat flour, water, salt, yeast. Watch out for bad oils and soy derivatives.

Barley, Kamut & Rye These are other gluten grains that can be used to make bread, although I've only had experience with Barley. They are all great to use, just be sure to prepare them properly

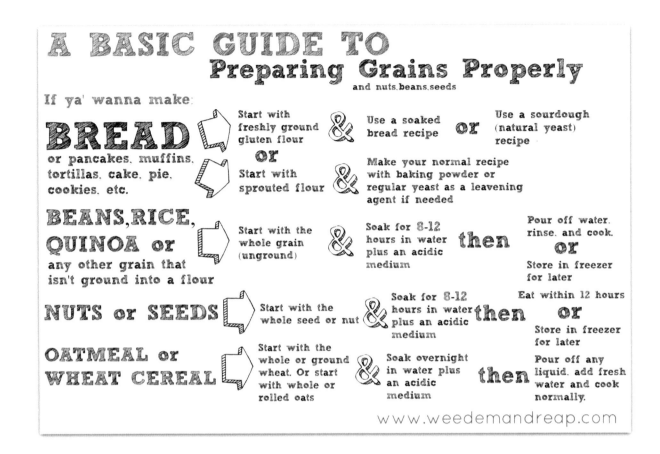

DAIRY

About four years ago, we made the switch as a family to raw milk. Knowing that traditional societies have thrived off raw dairy for years made us comfortable with our decision. Also, knowing that pasteurization was only invented after farms were making people sick from keeping cows in close confinement, made us feel even safer that our milk was coming from healthy, pasture-raised animals. Raw milk contains many amazing enzymes that actually kill pathogens if they should ever contaminate milk. Lacto-peroxidase, lacto-ferrin, anti-microbial cells, and healthy carbohydrates, a ton of healthy medium chain fatty acids, enzymes, vitamins, and minerals are all affected by pasteurization, and I want all that stuff in my milk! Raw milk stimulates the immune system, heals your gut, and ensures that all those nutrients are readily absorbed! While the CDC has held their stance against ingesting raw milk over the years, a recent quantitative risk assessment published by the Journal of Food Protection demonstrated that raw milk is a low-risk food. Since the 1930s (and the rise of factory farm/pasteurization), raw milk has been touted as unsafe, but this assessment determined, once and for all, that raw milk is low-risk. In fact, in this assessment they found that green leafy vegetables are the most frequent cause of food-borne illnesses.

We love drinking raw milk, and we've noticed some amazing health benefits, particularly with my son who used to have severe asthma. We purchased our own goats and milk them morning and night for fresh raw milk. For optimal health of the cow/goat/sheep and optimal nutrition of the milk, the animal needs its natural habitat.

Ruminant animals -- cattle, sheep, goats, buffalo, deer, elk, giraffes, and camels -- all depend on bacteria to digest their food for them. These animals technically don't obtain nutrition from their food. Instead, they rely on the bacteria to digest their food for them, and then the ruminant animal obtains their nutrition from the byproducts of the bacteria. It's actually an amazing process, and one we should all be thankful for, as 50% of the world's grasses & crops can only be digested by these kinds of animals. This is why we humans can't stick our faces in the grass and start chompin' away. We're not ruminant animals, so we depend on them to eat up that grass and provide milk and meat for us. It's actually an awesome "circle of life" concept if you think about it! (Cue Lion King soundtrack.) Just so we're clear, a ruminant animal doesn't have to be fed 100% pure grass to be healthy, it just needs grass as its primary source of nutrition. Ruminant animals also produce phytase, an enzyme that helps their bodies break down the blocking phytic acid in grains. Traditionally, farmers have been feeding animals grains for thousands of years, but only in small amounts. Grains were typically fed at the end of a crop harvest to "finish" an animal raised for meat, or in small amounts year-round at the milking stand. I would say an animal fed roughly 80% grass & 20% grains would be the max allowance of grains. It's even better if the grains being fed are organic.

The website www.realmilk.com is a fantastic resource for those searching for good, quality raw milk, and I'd even recommend searching Craigslist as well. No matter what, you should visit the farm and check out the living conditions and ask about the amounts of grass & grain. Finally, what to do if you can't find good quality, raw, grass-fed milk or if it's illegal in your state? First, you must understand that pasteurization is most harmful to the carrier proteins in the milk, while most of the fat-soluble vitamins are preserved, particularly Vitamins D, E, & K. Because of this, you can eat pasteurized butter & cream, and if you need milk, you can dilute the cream with filtered water. Also, because the carrier proteins are harder to digest, it would be best to culture your pasteurized dairy.

"If you cannot find good quality raw milk, you should limit your consumption of milk products to cultured milk, cultured buttermilk, whole milk yoghurt, butter, cream and raw cheeses."

- Sally Fallon

By sticking with cream you are avoiding two things: hard to digest denatured proteins and homogenization, which makes the proteins even harder to digest. Of course, the best is organic grass-fed milk, but not everybody has access to the best. So just for you, I've made a handy-dandy guide...

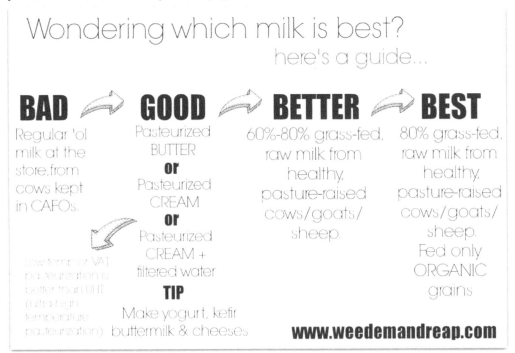

The most important thing is that you are eating WHOLE FAT dairy. Enjoy butter, cheese, milk, and yogurt and just do your best to find the highest-quality you can afford. When searching for raw milk, you can go to www.realmilk.com and search in the real milk finder box.

EGGS:

Cage-free. Free-range. Pasture-raised. If you're new to real food, then you'll need to know the difference between these titles. Why? Because all eggs ain't created equally. Ever since farmers started stuffing millions of chickens into teeny tiny living spaces and calling it "farm fresh," we as consumers have had to work hard to understand what it is we really are buying. Believe it or not, the nutritional quality of your eggs will depend on where your chickens get to chill out. Have you ever tasted a REAL farm fresh egg from a chicken that has had the opportunity to roam a pasture and to peck and scratch in the ground? I hadn't until a couple years ago when we started to raise chickens, and let me tell you...the taste of a REAL farm fresh egg is AMAZING!

Search for "pasture-raised" eggs, which mean the chickens have been able to live in an actual pasture with grass and bugs. "Cage-free" and "Free-range" are simply chickens allowed to roam, but still stuffed in a small space with other chickens.

MEATS

Again, try to find the highest quality. Grass-fed meat that is only finished on a small amount of grains is the best option. Next best would be meat labeled only "organic." Finally, if all you can find is hormone-free or antibiotic-free, often labeled "natural," you're still doing better than buying regular ol' meat with hormones & anti-biotics. **The most important thing is that you are buying meat in whole pieces, like a whole chicken, and that you aren't afraid of fats from meats.** By purchasing whole cuts of meats (with bones), you can make a healing bone broth, which will help stretch that budget of yours! Also, understand that meat doesn't have to be part of every single meal. We eat meat a couple times a week and use broth a couple times a week as well and call it good. You can read my extensive article on how to purchase grass-fed beef in bulk here! http://www.weedemandreap.com/2013/07/how-to-purchase-grass-fed-beef-in-bulk.html

SEAFOOD

You don't need to be afraid of the mercury in fish because seafood is also high in selenium, which binds with mercury and prevents your body from absorbing the mercury. Traditional societies have lived for centuries on the stuff, so don't let modern studies fool you. It is best, however, to look for "wild caught" varieties. Farm-raised fish just aren't as healthy and don't offer you the same health benefits. Also, since GMO salmon was just approved by the FDA, we need to focus more on real, wild seafood.

SWEETENERS

Choose from any of these sweeteners for your home cooking/baking:

• Local Honey
• Maple Syrup
• Stevia
• Unrefined brown cane sugar (such as Rapadura or Sucunat)
• Coconut sugar

FATS

The most important thing is to not be afraid of fats! Use butter, tallow, coconut oil, or olive oil liberally!

For HIGH HEAT cooking or FRYING:

Lard - We use lard to make crispy fried chicken, make deliciously flaky pies, and cook a simple food like eggs or hash browns. It's not smelly, it's divine! Food was meant to be enjoyed! And trust me, lard makes EVERYTHING taste a little better. Odds are, you are going to have the best luck finding pig fat, then rendering it yourself to make lard. Rendering lard is SUPER easy, and I've included a recipe at the end of this book. There are two kinds of pig fat: back fat & leaf (internal) fat. One of the most important things you'll need to find is a pork or meat shop that raises pigs who are pastured or foraged. This means they were able to be outside and soak up the sun - hence the reason why lard is so high in Vitamin D. It is also a general rule that animals are cleaner and healthier when they are allowed to be in their natural environment instead of a small dark cage surrounded by bajillions of other pigs.

Tallow – Tallow is the fat situated around the kidneys of beef & mutton/lamb. It is rendered just like lard, over low heat for about 6-8 hours, and then strained into mason jars and stored in the fridge.

Ghee – Ghee is clarified butter. Not only does it taste amazing, it also has a high smoke-point!

Coconut Oil – Great for cooking at moderately-high heats, coconut oil really compliments any dish! If you'd like to avoid that coconut flavor, purchase expeller-pressed instead of virgin. Look for coconut oil in bulk! We buy 1 gallon at Costco for $22.

For LOW HEAT cooking or sautéing:

Butter, butter, & more butter – We LOVE the Kerrygold brand butter. It's low-temp pasteurized, primarily grass-fed, deliciously rich butter.

Olive oil – extra-virgin cold pressed is best.

For NO HEAT applications like salad dressing or mayo:

Avocado oil - naturally refined or cold-pressed
Flaxseed, Walnut, Sesame, or Macadamia Nut oil – use in moderation

HOW TO AFFORD REAL FOOD

I spend about $400-$500 a month on groceries (family of four). That's without trying to stick to a budget. If I had to stick to a budget, I think I could get it down to $350 a month if I absolutely had to. My husband is seriously the most frugal man in the world, and it was definitely hard at first to convince him of the benefit of spending more money on healthy food! Just take your time, shop the sales, and remember…

"If you think organic food is expensive, have you priced cancer lately?"

*-**Joel** Salatin, Founder of Polyface Farms*

My husband now agrees with me that food is the most important expense that we have. It's become one of our first priorities, and thanks to real food, instead of spending $10,000 per year on health care (I was really sick ya'll), we now spend about $500.

"Is it just a coincidence that as the portion of our income spent on food has declined, spending on health care has soared? In 1960 Americans spent 17.5 percent of their income on food and 5.2 percent of national income on health care. Since then, those numbers have flipped: Spending on food has fallen to 9.9 percent, while spending on health care has climbed to 16 percent of national income. I have to think that by spending a little more on healthier food we could reduce the amount we have to spend on health care."

*-**Michael Pollan**, In Defense of Food: An Eater's Manifesto*

MORE BUDGET-SAVING TIPS

Start a vegetable garden – You'd be surprised how much you can grow in a tiny amount of space!

Shop in Bulk – My favorite company to shop in bulk is Azure Standard. They deliver almost anywhere and have great prices. Costco is beginning to carry some good organic food as well like peanut butter, jam, grains, Kerrygold butter, and grass-fed meat.

Avoid Expensive Organic Packaged Food – This is a common mistake new real foodies make. You'll want to avoid this because it really upsets your budget, and it's really not optimal food anyway.

THE BIGGEST MISTAKE NEW REAL FOODIES MAKE:

When I first became a real foodist, I was motivated. Boy, was I motivated! I made homemade poptarts and fruit leather and fishy crackers (yes in the shape of fishies complete with a smiley face), and I effectively trapped myself in real food HELL. I noticed that I became strangely protective of my homemade goodies. I began to get mad if anybody ate them. I hid them so we wouldn't eat them so fast. Ironic, huh? And, in the end, I decided it was just too much work for this busy momma.

Don't get me wrong, it's not like those homemade goodies aren't healthy. They are! And props to you if you have the time to make them. But here's what I've found and what I tell everybody about real food: It's not about recreating every single dang dog snack in the grocery store. It's about eating REAL FOOD. Here's the thing; processed food is made in a factory. With probably like 100 or so workers. And franken-crazy ingredients. So, just accept the fact that you're not going to be able to recreate Wheat Thins and Fruit Roll-ups and Doritos and Trix-flavored Go-gurts. It ain't gonna happen.

But do you know what the most amazing thing about real food is? Once you start feeding your family real, nourishing food, you'll find they don't snack. Hardly ever. It's really spectacular how much we all used to snack and snack all day, and now it's such a rare occurrence. If we get hungry, we'll have one snack in the afternoon, but usually it's something simple like fruit or cheese or nuts. And let me tell you, it makes my life blissfully easier. So, take it from me, if you're feeling overwhelmed at the thought of having to become that homemade mommy, just relax. I just took a huge load off your shoulders. Just make balanced, nourishing meals 3 times a day, and call it good.

THE GOOD-BETTER-BEST PRINCIPLE

Remember the good-better-best principle. Don't give up if you can't buy everything organic and grass-fed! The most important thing is that you are avoiding processed foods (fruit snacks, granola bars, cereal, cookies, crackers, chips, soda, etc.) and focusing on REAL FOOD! I promise you will see a difference once you start turning away from processed foods. Live the 80/20 rule and enjoy life while losing weight!

THE REAL FOOD GOOD-BETTER-BEST PRINCIPLE

"DOING THE BEST YOU CAN WITH WHAT YOU HAVE"

	BAD	GOOD	BETTER	BEST
FRUITS & VEGETABLES	NOT EATING ANY FRESH FRUITS or VEGETABLES	BUYING ONLY CONVENTIONAL FRUITS and VEGETABLES	USING THE DIRTY DOZEN CLEAN FIFTEEN RULE & BUYING ORGANIC WHEN AFFORDABLE	BUYING ALL ORGANIC, LOCAL & SEASONAL or GROWING YOUR OWN
GRAINS, BEANS NUTS & SEEDS	OBTAINING THEM ONLY FROM PACKAGED CEREALS, CRACKERS, CHIPS GRANOLA BARS, & SNACK FOODS	HOMEMADE COOKING WITH SOME REFINED FLOURS & SOME WHOLE GRAIN FLOUR, BEANS, NUTS, & SEEDS	HOMEMADE COOKING WITH ALL 100% WHOLE GRAIN FLOURS & GRAINS	HOMEMADE COOKING WITH ALL 100% WHOLE GRAINS & PREPARING PROPERLY BY SOAKING, SPROUTING, or SOUR LEAVENING
EGGS	EATING EGG WHITES ONLY, POWDERED EGGS, or OTHER EGG-LIKE PRODUCTS	BUYING CONVENTIONAL STOREBOUGHT EGGS	BUYING STOREBOUGHT ORGANIC, FREE-RANGE EGGS	BUYING ORGANIC & LOCAL PASTURE-RAISED EGGS
DAIRY	LOW-FAT DAIRY PRODUCTS, *CAFO MILK PRODUCTS or HIGH-TEMP PASTEURIZED	WHOLE DAIRY, PRIMARILY GRASS-FED & LOW-TEMP PASTEURIZED	WHOLE DAIRY, PRIMARILY GRASS-FED & RAW	WHOLE DAIRY, PRIMARILY GRASS-FED, PASTURE-RAISED, ORGANIC & RAW
MEAT	BONELESS, SKINLESS MEAT, *CAFO MEAT or OTHER MEAT-LIKE PRODUCTS	WHOLE MEAT ANTI-BIOTIC & HORMONE FREE	WHOLE MEAT GRASS-FED and/or ORGANIC	WHOLE MEAT, PRIMARILY GRASS-FED and/or ORGANIC & PASTURE-RAISED
SEAFOOD	GENETICALLY MODIFIED or SEAFOOD-LIKE PRODUCTS	FARM-RAISED SEAFOOD	BPA-FREE CANNED or FROZEN WILD-CAUGHT SEAFOOD	FRESH & LOCAL WILD-CAUGHT SEAFOOD
FATS	MARGARINE, CRISCO, SOYBEAN OIL CORN, CANOLA, VEGETABLE or HYDROGENATED OILS	PASTEURIZED STORE BOUGHT GRAIN-FED BUTTER	PASTEURIZED ORGANIC GRASS-FED BUTTER or REGULAR COCONUT or OLIVE OIL	GRASS-FED LARD & TALLOW or ORGANIC, EXTRA-VIRGIN COCONUT or OLIVE OIL / RAW BUTTER
SWEETENERS	HIGH FRUCTOSE CORN SYRUP, REGULAR, GMO SUGAR, or SUGAR SUBSTITUTES	100% PURE WHITE UNREFINED CANE SUGAR	UNREFINED CANE SUGAR or STORE BOUGHT HONEY or REAL MAPLE SYRUP	LOCAL HONEY or ORGANIC UNREFINED CANE SUGAR or ORGANIC REAL MAPLE SYRUP / PURE STEVIA or COCONUT SUGAR
PANTRY ITEMS	REGULAR, STOREBOUGHT *GMO LADEN CEREALS, CRACKERS, CHIPS GRANOLA BARS, & SNACK FOODS	ORGANIC, NON-GMO CEREALS, CRACKERS, CHIPS GRANOLA BARS, & SNACK FOODS	HOMEMADE, WHOLE GRAIN CEREALS, CRACKERS, CHIPS GRANOLA BARS, & FRUIT SNACKS	HOMEMADE, WHOLE GRAIN *PROPERLY PREPARED SNACK FOODS or STOP RE-CREATING THEM ALTOGETHER.
FRIDGE ITEMS	REGULAR, STOREBOUGHT *GMO LADEN SODA, JUICE, SNACK FOODS & CONDIMENTS	ORGANIC, NON-GMO SODA, JUICE, SNACK FOODS & CONDIMENTS	HOMEMADE SNACK FOODS & CONDIMENTS	HOMEMADE & PROPERLY PREPARED "SODA" aka WATER KEFIR or KOMBUCHA & *LACTO-FERMENTED CONDIMENTS

* CAFO - Concentrated Animal Feeding Operation
* PROPERLY PREPARED - By soaking, sprouting, or sour leavening the grains, nuts, beans, seeds
* LACTO-FERMENTED - Fermenting condiments as another source of homemade probiotics.

HOW TO TURN ANY RECIPE INTO A REAL FOOD MEAL:

While researching for real food recipes is an awesome endeavor, also remember that ANY recipe you currently cook with can be turned into a healthy, real food meal! Simply substitute the bad stuff for the good stuff and you're set!

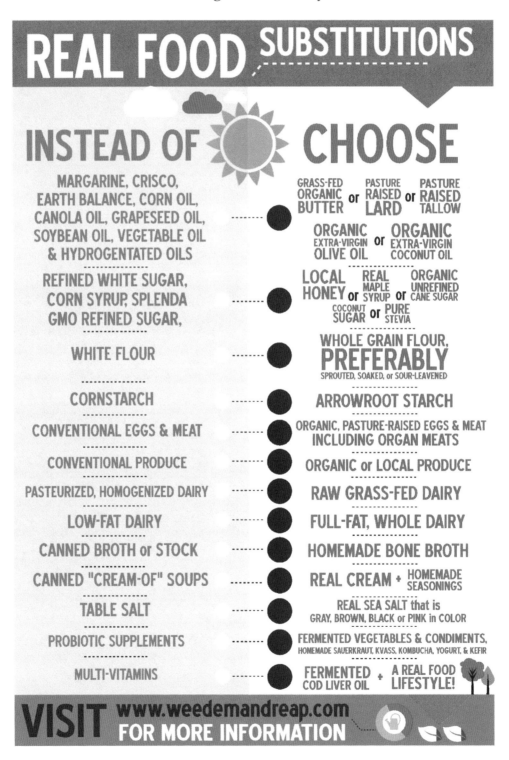

REAL FOOD
MEAL PLANS

WEEK ONE

MEALS	SUNDAY	MONDAY	TUESDAY	WEDNESDAY	THURSDAY	FRIDAY	SATURDAY
BREAKFAST	•Eggs, bacon, whole grain {soaked} biscuits, whole milk.	•Homemade yogurt with berries & leftover biscuits.	•Oatmeal {soaked} with nuts & maple syrup.	•Veggie omelets with buttered toast, whole milk.	•Homemade yogurt with berries & peanut butter toast.	•Sausage, fried eggs, •Sweet Potato Hash.	•Fruit smoothie with a handful of spinach, raw egg yolk, & powdered gelatin.
LUNCH	•Fresh garden salad with homemade ranch dressing.	•Egg salad Sandwich or wrap, veggies & fruit	•Tuna salad sandwich, leftover coleslaw	•Leftover Cheesy Broccoli Soup	•Grilled cheese sandwiches, tomato soup.	•Leftover Salmon, cheese quesadilla with corn {organic sprouted} tortillas	•PB & J Sandwiches OR leftover Pizza & Soda
DINNER	•Slow-cooker Pot Roast w/ red potatoes & carrots. •Homemade gravy.	•BBQ Beef Sandwiches •Homemade coleslaw.	•Cheesy Broccoli Soup	•Tostadas with corn tortillas {organic sprouted} refried beans, cheese, tomatoes.	•Honey-Glazed Salmon •Baked Sweet Potatoes.	•Homemade Pizza & Homemade soda	•Grassfed Hotdogs & Potato Chips OR Out-to-eat
DESSERT	•Whole Grain Brownies			•Blueberry Lemon Gelato			

Week ONE – "THE BREAKDOWN" (with prep times)

The night before: (20 min) {soak} Whole-Grain Biscuits, {start} Homemade Yogurt. {defrost} roast **Sunday morning**: (30 min) {bake} biscuits, {cook} Scrambled Eggs & bacon, {start} Roast, Potatoes & Carrots in crockpot, {prepare} Ranch Dressing, (refrigerate) leftover yogurt
Sunday afternoon: (5 min) {make} lunch (fresh garden salad) and eat with dressing, {make} hard boiled eggs, then refrigerate
Sunday evening: (20 min) {remove & slice} roast to let cool, {make} Homemade Gravy & {make} Whole-Grain Brownies

The night before: (2 min) {refrigerate} leftover roast, {store} brownies to go with lunches
Monday morning: (15 min) Make breakfast (yogurt, berries, leftover biscuits), {prepare} Egg Salad & refrigerate
Monday afternoon: Eat lunch (egg salad, fruits, veggies)
Monday evening: (20 min) {re-heat} leftover roast w/ Homemade BBQ Sauce. {make} Coleslaw.

The night before: (5 min) {start} Homemade Bone Broth with bones from roast in crockpot to cook 18- 24 hours, {soak} Oatmeal
Tuesday morning: (20 min) {cook} oatmeal, {prepare} Tuna Salad & refrigerate
Tuesday afternoon: Eat lunch (tuna salad & leftover coleslaw)
Tuesday evening: (30 min) {make} Cheesy Potato Broccoli Soup with bone broth, {freeze} leftover broth for next week.

The night before: (5 min) {refrigerate} leftover soup, {soak} beans for Refried Beans,
Wednesday morning: (10 min) {make} breakfast (veggie omelets), {start} beans in crockpot.
Wednesday afternoon: Eat lunch (leftover soup)
Wednesday evening: (30 min) {finish} beans, {fry} tortillas in traditional oil, {prepare} toppings. {make} Blueberry Lemon Gelato

The night before: (15 min) {start} Homemade Yogurt (if you don't have enough leftovers from Monday)
Thursday morning: (30 min) {make} breakfast (yogurt, berries, & PB toast), {start} Homemade Soda.
Thursday afternoon: (15 min) {make} lunch (Grilled Cheese Sandwiches & store bought organic tomato soup)
Thursday evening: (45 min) {make} Honey–Glazed Salmon & Baked Sweet Potatoes.

The night before: (10 min) {refrigerate} leftover salmon & sweet potatoes, {bottle} soda
Friday morning: (20 min) {make} Sweet Potato Hash, fried eggs, & sausage (MSG-free, natural/organic) {refrigerate} soda
Friday afternoon: (15 min) {make} lunch (quesadillas with corn tortillas, cheese, & any leftover salmon),
Friday evening: (45min) {make} Homemade Pizza

The night before: nothing
Saturday morning: (10 min) {make} breakfast (smoothies)
Saturday afternoon: (15 min) {make} lunch (PB sandwiches or leftover pizza)
Saturday evening: (10min) Grass-fed Hotdogs & natural/organic potato chips OR Out-to-eat

Week ONE –"THE GROCERY LIST" (FOR 6 PEOPLE)

GROCERY STORE/FARMER'S MARKET

- 4 dozen eggs (organic)
- 1 lb. bacon (MSG-free, uncured)
- 1 lb. sausage (MSG-free, uncured)
- Grass-fed/organic hot dogs
- 2 lb. Wild-caught Salmon
- (2) 3-4 lb. rump roast
- 5 lb. red potatoes
- 8 russet potatoes
- 6-8 sweet potatoes
- 2 lb. carrots, 2 onions
- 1 head celery, 1 cucumber
- 2 head lettuce (any variety)
- 1 small bunch spinach
- 4 tomatoes, 4 avocados
- 1-2 Veggies (any) for lunches
- 1 Fruit (any) for lunches
- 1 bag coleslaw mix
- 2 apples, 8 oz. berries (any)
- 2 head broccoli, bananas
- bottled organic juice (not citrus)
- 2 pkg. Sprouted/organic corn tortillas
- 3 loaves Bread (whole-grain or sprouted)
- 2.5 lb. cheddar cheese
- 1 lb. mozzarella cheese
- Organic tomato soup
- Jarred marinara sauce (for pizza)
- Pizza Toppings of your choice
- Natural/organic potato chips
- 2-4 gallons whole milk (preferably raw & grass fed)
- I pint cream, 16 oz. sour cream

PANTRY

- Whole-wheat, Spelt, Emer, or Einkhorn flour (sprouted is even better)
- Rolled Oats
- Dried Pinto Beans
- Salt (sea or celtic)
- Baking Soda & Baking Powder
- Homemade Ranch Mix
- Organic Cornstarch
- Powdered Cocoa
- Unrefined sweetener (brown cane sugar, coconut sugar, honey, maple syrup)
- Real Vanilla
- Coconut Oil, Lard, or Tallow
- Olive Oil
- Tomato Paste
- Natural Liquid Smoke (optional)
- 2 cans Wild-Caught Tuna
- Powdered Grass-fed Gelatin
- Onion, garlic, chili, cayenne powder, thyme

FRIDGE/FREEZER

- Butter (preferably grass-fed)
- Powdered Yogurt Starter
- Organic Mayonnaise
- Organic Mustard
- Molasses
- Apple Cider Vinegar
- Pureed, frozen liver
- Chicken, Beef, or Lamb Bones (for broth)
- Water kefir grains
- Organic Peanut Butter
- Organic Jam
- 1 c. walnuts/pecans
- Active dry yeast

WEEK TWO

MEALS	SUNDAY	MONDAY	TUESDAY	WEDNESDAY	THURSDAY	FRIDAY	SATURDAY
BREAKFAST	•Whole-grain {sprouted} flour pancakes, fried eggs, fruit.	•Homemade yogurt with fruit & {soaked} nuts.	•Leftover pancakes with full-fat cream cheese & jam	•Omelets with veggies & cheese, fruit.	•Oatmeal {soaked} with nuts & maple syrup.	•Peanut butter & banana smoothie with whole milk, raw egg yolk, gelatin.	•Bacon & eggs, fried potatoes, fresh fruit
LUNCH	•Grilled Cheese Sandwiches, veggies & fruit.	•Leftover meatloaf bites w/ mashed potatoes & fresh veggies.	•Cobb Salad with bacon, boiled eggs, tomatoes, carrots, avocado & homemade ranch dressing.	•Leftover chili & cornbread	•PB & J Sandwiches, Cream cheese & apple sandwiches, & veggies.	•Leftover sweet n' sour chicken w/ rice & fresh veggies.	•Leftover homemade pizza OR Egg salad sandwiches
DINNER	•Meatloaf w/ Perfect Mashed Potatoes & buttered green beans.	•Veggie Lasagna, fresh garden salad with homemade ranch dressing.	•Classic Beef Chili with {soaked} cornbread	•Loaded Baked Potates with steamed, buttered broccoli.	•Sweet n' Sour Chicken with organic steamed rice & steamed, buttered zucchini	•Homemade Pizza & homemade soda	•Homemade Mac n' Cheese OR Out-to-eat
DESSERT	•Homemade Chocolate Chip Cookies			•Homemade Ice Cream			

Week TWO – "THE BREAKDOWN" (with prep times)

The night before: nothing
Sunday morning: (30 min) {make} Whole-Grain Sprouted Pancakes, eggs, fruit {defrost} ground beef
Sunday afternoon: (15 min) {make} lunch (Grilled Cheese Sandwiches, veggies & fruit)
Sunday evening: (30 min) {make} Meatloaf & Perfect Mashed Potatoes, green beans, {make} Homemade Chocolate Chip Cookies

The night before: (15 min) {soak} nuts, {start} Homemade Yogurt {store} leftovers
Monday morning: (5 min) {make} breakfast (yogurt, nuts, fruit), {mix} Homemade Ranch Dressing, {refrigerate} leftover yogurt
Monday afternoon: (5 min) {re-heat} leftover lunch (meatloaf, potatoes, veggies)
Monday evening: (20 min) {make} Veggie Lasagna, garden salad

The night before: (5 min) {soak} beans {soak} cornbread,
Tuesday morning: (20 min) {make} breakfast (leftover pancakes), {start} Classic Chili in crockpot, {make} hard boiled eggs
Tuesday afternoon: (10 min) {make} Cobb salad
Tuesday evening: (15 min) {make} Cornbread

The night before: nothing
Wednesday morning: (10 min) {make} breakfast (omelets with veggies, fruit)
Wednesday afternoon: (5 min) {re-heat} lunch (leftover chili & cornbread)
Wednesday evening: (30) {make} Baked Potatoes (make extra for Saturday morning hash browns), {steam} broccoli, {cook} bacon, {make} Homemade Ice Cream

The night before: (2 min) {soak} Oatmeal, {soak} nuts.
Thursday morning: (10 min) {make} breakfast (oatmeal, nuts), {defrost} chicken, {start} Homemade Soda.
Thursday afternoon: (15 min) {make} lunch (PB&J sandwiches, Cream Cheese Apple Sandwiches, veggies)
Thursday evening: (45 min) {make} Sweet n' Sour Chicken, {cook} Steamed Rice & zucchini

The night before: {bottle} soda
Friday morning: (10 min) {make} PB banana smoothie, {refrigerate} soda
Friday afternoon: (5 min) {re-heat} lunch (leftover sweet n' sour chicken & rice)
Friday evening: (45min) {make} Homemade Pizza

The night before: nothing
Saturday morning: (20 min) {make} breakfast (bacon, eggs, fruit)
Saturday afternoon: (15 min) {re-heat} lunch (leftover pizza) or egg salad sandwiches
Saturday evening: (30min) {make} Homemade Mac n' Cheese OR Out-to-eat

Week TWO – "THE GROCERY LIST" (FOR 6 PEOPLE)

GROCERY STORE/FARMER'S MARKET
- 3 dozen eggs (organic)
- 1 lb. bacon (MSG-free, uncured)
- 2-3 lb. chicken (breasts, thighs, tenderloins – with skin)
- 3 lb. ground beef
- 5 lb. red potatoes
- 5 lb. russet potatoes
- 2 lb. carrots
- 6 medium tomatoes
- 2 avocados
- 1 onion, 1 head celery
- 2 head lettuce (any variety)
- 4 medium zucchinis
- 1-2 Veggies (any) for lunches
- 2 Fruit (any) for lunch/breakfast
- 3 apples, 1 bunch bananas
- 1 fruit for ice cream
- 1 head broccoli
- 1 lb. green beans
bottled organic juice (not citrus)
- 1 lb. cheddar cheese
- 1 lb. mozzarella cheese
- 2 Jars marinara sauce (for lasagna & pizza)
- Pizza Toppings of your choice
- 2-4 gallons whole milk (preferably raw & grass fed)
- 2 loaves bread (whole grain or sprouted)
- 16 oz. cream cheese
- 1 pint heavy cream

PANTRY
- Whole-wheat, Spelt, Emer, or Einkhorn flour (sprouted is even better)
- Rolled Oats
- Dried Pinto Beans
- Dried Kidney Beans
- White Jasmine or Basmati Rice
- Salt (sea or celtic)
- Baking Powder
- Homemade Ranch Mix
- Homemade Taco Seasoning
- Organic Cornstarch
- Arrowroot Starch
- Unrefined sweetener (brown cane sugar, coconut sugar, honey, maple syrup)
- Real Vanilla
- Coconut Oil, Lard, or Tallow
- Olive Oil
- 1 can BPA-free tomato sauce
- 1 can BPA-free tomato paste
- Powdered Grass-fed Gelatin

FRIDGE/FREEZER
- Butter (preferably grass-fed)
- Powdered Yogurt Starter
- Organic Mayonnaise
- Organic Ketchup
- Organic Mustard
- Apple Cider Vinegar
- Chili powder, garlic powder
- Pureed, frozen liver
- Water kefir grains
- Organic Peanut Butter
- Organic Jam
- Coconut Aminos (soy sauce)
- 2 c. walnuts/pecans
- Active dry yeast
- Broth (stored from last week)

WEEK THREE

MEALS	SUNDAY	MONDAY	TUESDAY	WEDNESDAY	THURSDAY	FRIDAY	SATURDAY
BREAKFAST	●Whole-Grain Sprouted Waffles w/ maple syrup, eggs.	●Homemade yogurt with fruit & {soaked} granola.	●Omelets with veggies & cheese, fruit.	●Granola {soaked} with whole milk, fresh fruit.	●Sausage, fried eggs, & toast.	●Oatmeal {soaked} with nuts & maple syrup.	●Fruit smoothie with a handful of spinach, raw egg yolk, & powdered gelatin.
LUNCH	●Waldorf salad w/ greens, apples, pecans, blue cheese, & vinagrette.	●Grilled Cheese Sandwiches, veggies & fruit.	●Cheese Quesadillas made with whole-grain {soaked} tortillas.	●Chicken salad sandwiches , fresh fruit & veggies.	●Leftover chicken noodle soup	●Tuna salad sandwich, fresh veggies & fruit.	●Leftover pizza & soda
DINNER	●Perfect Grilled Steak w/ smashed potatoes & parmesan broccoli	●Fajitas (leftover steak) with whole-grain {soaked} tortillas ● Mexican Rice	●Slow-cooker Chicken noodle soup	●Navajo Tacos with beans, cheese, lettuce, & salsa.	●Fish n' Chips w/ homemade coleslaw.	●Homemade Pizza & homemade soda	●Ultimate Nachos OR Out-to-eat
DESSERT	●Homemade Donuts			●Leftover Navajo Taco Fry Bread with honey			

Week THREE – "THE BREAKDOWN" (with prep times)

The night before: (10 min) {soak} granola
Sunday morning: (30 min) {make} Whole-grain Sprouted Waffles {soak} donuts, {dehydrate} granola
Sunday afternoon: (15 min) {make} lunch (Waldorf Salad)
Sunday evening: (45 min) {make} Perfect Grilled Steak& Smashed Potatoes, Parmesan Broccoli, {make} Homemade Donuts

The night before: (15 min) {soak} nuts, {start} Homemade Yogurt, {store} granola in airtight container.
Monday morning: (5 min) {make} breakfast (yogurt, granola, fruit), {refrigerate} leftover yogurt, {soak} tortillas {start} Homemade Bone Broth
Monday afternoon: (5 min) {make} lunch Grilled Cheese Sandwiches, veggies & fruit
Monday evening: (40 min) {make} Fajitas, Homemade Tortillas, & Cheesy Mexican Rice

The night before: (10 min)
Tuesday morning: (20 min) {make} breakfast, (omelets with veggies & cheese, fruit) {start} Chicken Noodle Soup in crockpot
Tuesday afternoon: (10 min) {make} lunch (cheese quesadillas, veggies, fruit)
Tuesday evening: (5 min) {finish} chicken noodle soup, {reserve} half of cooked chicken for next day's lunch.

The night before: (5 min) {refrigerate} leftover soup, {refrigerate} cooked chicken, {soak} beans, {soak} Navajo Taco dough
Wednesday morning: (10 min) {make} breakfast (granola, milk, fruit), {start} beans in crockpot.
Wednesday afternoon: (10 min) {make} Chicken Salad Sandwiches
Wednesday evening: (45 min) {make} Fresh n' Easy Salsa, {finish} Refried Beans, {fry} navajo tacos

The night before: nothing
Thursday morning: (10 min) {make} breakfast (sausage, fried eggs, toast), {start} Homemade Soda
Thursday afternoon: (15 min) {re-heat} lunch (leftover soup)
Thursday evening: (45 min) {make} Coleslaw, {cook} Fish n' Chips

The night before: {soak} Oatmeal, {bottle} soda
Friday morning: (10 min) {make} breakfast (oatmeal, nuts,), {refrigerate} soda
Friday afternoon: (5 min) {make} lunch (Tuna Salad sandwiches)
Friday evening: (45min) {make} Homemade Pizza

The night before: nothing
Saturday morning: (20 min) {make} breakfast (fruit smoothies)
Saturday afternoon: (15 min) {re-heat} leftover lunch
Saturday evening: (30min) {make} Ultimate Nachos OR Out-to-eat

Week THREE – "THE GROCERY LIST" (FOR 6 PEOPLE)

GROCERY STORE/FARMER'S MARKET

- 3 dozen eggs (organic)
- 4-6 beef steaks
- 1 lb. ground beef
- (2) 2 lb. half chicken
- 6 codfish filets
- 6-8 russet potatoes
- 6-8 red potatoes
- 1 head broccoli
- 1-2 Veggies (any) for lunches
- 2 Fruit (any) for lunch/breakfast
- 2 pkg. organic/sprouted corn tortillas
- 1 bulb garlic, 2 onions
- 2 lb. mixed greens
- 4 apples, 1 bunch grapes
- 1 lb. carrots, 1 head celery
- 1 bunch green onions
- 4 tomatoes, 1 bunch cilantro
- 1 pint cream
- 3 lb. cheddar cheese
- 2 lb. mozzarella cheese
- 6 oz. parmesan cheese
- 6 oz. blue cheese (or feta)
- v2-4 gallons whole milk (preferably raw & grass fed)
- 1 bag coleslaw mix
- 1 jars marinara sauce (for pizza)
- Pizza Toppings of your choice
- 2 loaves bread (whole grain or sprouted)
- 2 bags organic tortilla chips

PANTRY

- Whole-wheat, Spelt, Emer, or Einkhorn flour (sprouted is even better)
- Whole Oats
- Dried Pinto Beans
- White Jasmine or Basmati Rice
- 1 pkg. pasta (organic or sprouted)
- Bread Crumbs
- Salt (sea or celtic)
- Baking Soda & Baking Powder
- Homemade Ranch Mix
- Homemade Taco Seasoning
- Homemade Italian Seasoning
- Organic Cornstarch
- Arrowroot Starch
- Powdered Cocoa
- Unrefined sweetener (brown cane sugar, coconut sugar, honey, maple syrup)
- Real Vanilla
- Coconut Oil, Lard, or Tallow
- Olive Oil
- Tomato Paste
- Wild-Caught Canned Tuna
- Powdered Grass-fed Gelatin
- 1 can organic coconut milk
- 1 can green chilies

FRIDGE/FREEZER

- Butter (preferably grass-fed)
- Powdered Yogurt Starter
- Organic Mayonnaise
- Organic Mustard
- Apple Cider Vinegar
- Chili powder
- Chicken, Beef, or Lamb Bones (for broth)
- Water kefir grains
- Organic Peanut Butter
- Organic Jam
- 2 c. walnuts/pecans
- Active dry yeast

WEEK FOUR

MEALS	SUNDAY	MONDAY	TUESDAY	WEDNESDAY	THURSDAY	FRIDAY	SATURDAY
BREAKFAST	●Whole-grain crepes with whipped cream & fresh strawberries & bananas, fried eggs.	●Sausage, eggs, & sweet potato hash.	●Oatmeal {soaked} with nuts & maple syrup.	●Omelets with veggies & cheese, fruit.	●Homemade yogurt with almond butter & jelly.	●Scrambled eggs, toast, whole milk, banana.	●Peanut butter & banana smoothie with whole milk, raw egg yolk, gelatin.
LUNCH	●Hummus & Corn {organic} chips, fruit & cheese platter.	●Grilled cheese sandwiches, tomato soup.	●Leftover enchiladas & salad.	●Leftover soup & rolls.	●Egg salad Sandwich or lettuce wrap, veggies & fruit	●Leftover Salmon patties & mango quinoa salad.	●Turkey {organic} sandwiches with cheese,tomato, lettuce. Fruit.
DINNER	●Roast Chicken w/ roasted root veggies	●Enchiladas w/ leftover chicken, corn {sprouted organic} tortillas, & fresh garden salad with homemade	●Roasted Butternut Squash Parmesan soup, ● Quick Sprouted Rolls	●Asian Lettuce Wraps & Asian Stir-fry	●Salmon Patties & Mango Quinoa Salad	●Homemade Pizza & homemade soda	●Hamburgers, potato salad, fruit OR Go Out-to-eat
DESSERT	●Homemade Cupcakes			●Homemade Fudgcicles			

Week FOUR – "THE BREAKDOWN" (with prep times)

The night before: (2 min) {defrost} 1 lb. chicken
Sunday morning: (20 min) {make} breakfast (crepes, eggs)
Sunday afternoon: (5 min) {make} lunch (hummus, chips, fruit, cheese)
Sunday evening: (40 min) {make} dinner (Roast Chicken, Roasted Root Vegetables)+ Baked Sweet Potatoes {make} Cupcakes

The night before: (2 min) {refrigerate} leftover chicken & sweet potatoes {start} yogurt {save} chicken bones
Monday morning: (15 min) {make} breakfast (sausage, eggs, Sweet Potato Hash) {make & refrigerate} Homemade Ranch Dressing
Monday afternoon: (15 min){make} lunch (Grilled Cheese Sandwiches, tomato soup)
Monday evening: (20 min) {make} dinner Chicken Enchiladas & garden salad w/ homemade ranch dressing, {start} Homemade Bone Broth

The night before: (5 min) {refrigerate} leftovers, {soak} Oatmeal, {soak} nuts,
Tuesday morning: (10 min) {make} breakfast (oatmeal, nuts, maple syrup, etc.)
Tuesday afternoon: (10 min) {make} lunch (leftover enchiladas & salad)
Tuesday evening: (45 min) {make} Roasted Butternut Squash Soup & Quick Sprouted Rolls

The night before: (5 min) {defrost} 1 lb. chicken {make} Homemade Fudge-sicles
Wednesday morning: (10 min) {make} breakfast (omelets w/ veggies, fruit)
Wednesday afternoon: (5 min) {re-heat} leftover soup & rolls
Wednesday evening: (45 min) {make} Asian Lettuce Wraps, Asian Stir-fry

The night before: (15 min) {start} yogurt, {soak} black beans {make} hard-boiled eggs
Thursday morning: (30 min) {make} breakfast (PB & J yogurt) {soak} quinoa
Thursday afternoon: (15 min) {make} lunch (Egg Salad, veggies, fruit) {cook, then refrigerate} black beans & quinoa
NSTRUCTIONS – How to cook quinoa can be found at: http://www.eatnakednow.com/tasty-tip-for-light-and-fluffy-quinoa/
 How to cook black beans can be found at:
http://www.homemademommy.net/2012/09/homemade-black-beans.html
Thursday evening: (45 min) {make} Mango Quinoa Salad, Salmon Patties

The night before: (5 min) {refrigerate} leftovers
Friday morning: (15 min) {make} breakfast (Scrambled Eggs, toast, milk, banana)
Friday afternoon: (5 min) {re-heat} leftovers (salmon patties & mango quinoa salad)
Friday evening: (45min) {make} Homemade Pizza

The night before: nothing
Saturday morning: (10 min) {make} breakfast (smoothies)
Saturday afternoon: (10 min) {re-heat} leftovers or {make} turkey sandwiches
Saturday evening: (30 min) {grill} hamburgers, {make} Potato Salad

Week FOUR – "THE GROCERY LIST"- (FOR 6 PEOPLE)

GROCERY STORE/FARMER'S MARKET

- 4 dozen eggs
- 1 quart cream
- 2 bunch bananas
- 1 16 oz. tub hummus
- 2 bag organic tortilla chips
- 1-2 whole chickens
- 1 lb. sausage
- 1 lb. organic turkey lunchmeat
- 3 lb. ground beef
- 5lb. russet potatoes
- 2 lb. assorted root veggies (potatoes, turnips, carrots, turnips)
- 2-3 sweet potatoes
- organic tomato soup
- 1 lb. cheddar cheese
- 2 heads lettuce, 2 tomatoes
- Fresh garden salad toppings
- 2 butternut squash
- 8 oz. parmesan cheese
- 2 c. bean sprouts
- 2 red & 1 yellow pepper
- 3 onions, 1 bunch green onions
- 2 mangos, 1 lime, 1 lemon
- 1 bunch cilantro, 2 clove garlic
- 1 jars marinara sauce (for pizza)
- Pizza Toppings of your choice
- 1 lb. mozzarella cheese
- 2-4 gallons whole milk (preferably raw & grass fed)
- 2 loaves bread

PANTRY

- Whole-wheat, Spelt, Emer, or Einkhorn flour (sprouted is even better)
- Whole Oats
- Potato Flakes
- White Quinoa
- Bread Crumbs
- Salt (sea or celtic)
- Baking Soda & Baking Powder
- Homemade Ranch Mix
- Organic Cornstarch
- Arrowroot Starch
- Powdered Cocoa
- Unrefined sweetener (brown cane sugar, coconut sugar, honey, maple syrup)
- Real Vanilla
- Coconut Oil, Lard, or Tallow
- Olive Oil
- Tomato Paste
- Canned Salmon
- Canned water chestnuts
- 1 can coconut milk
- Powdered Grass-fed Gelatin

FRIDGE/FREEZER

- Butter
- Powdered Yogurt Starter
- Organic Mayonnaise
- Organic Mustard
- Molasses
- Apple Cider Vinegar
- Dill weed, celery salt, thyme, oregano
- Chicken, Beef, or Lamb Bones (for broth)
- Coconut Aminos
- Water kefir grains
- Organic Peanut Butter or Almond Butter
- Organic Jam
- Active dry yeast

REAL FOOD RECIPES

The Basics

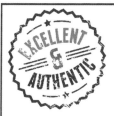

HOMEMADE RENDERED LARD or TALLOW

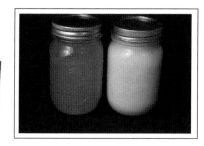

INGREDIENTS:

- 5 lbs. of pig fat (leaf or back fat) for LARD
OR
- 5 lbs. of beef suet (fat around the kidneys) for TALLOW
- 1 c. water

- big ol' pot
- colander
- thin dishtowel

DIRECTIONS:

1. Cut the fat into small 1-2 inch chunks. Place into a pot, add water and cook over low heat about 10-12 hours.
2. Strain the liquid fat away from the solid fat about 2-3 times throughout the cooking time. Let the strained liquid cool slowly on counter in jars.
3. When no more liquid is rendering from solid chunks, you are done.
4. Discard any leftover solid chunks.

5. The LARD or TALLOW will be a rich yellow color when hot, and as it cools, it will be come white.

MAKES 4 PINTS of LARD or TALLOW

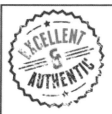

EASY BONE BROTH

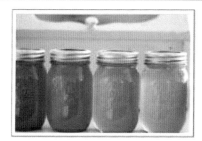

INGREDIENTS:

- 3 carrots
- 2 stalks celery
- 1/2 onion
- 2-3 chicken, beef, or lamb bones *
- 1/4 tsp. dried thyme
- 8 c. filtered water

*Roast bones for 1 hour at 350 before making broth.

CROCKPOT DIRECTIONS:

1. Chop vegetables into large chunks.
2. Place all ingredients in a crockpot
3. Cook on low for 12-24 hours.
4. Strain mixture through a dishtowel-lined colander.
5. Pour broth into mason jars and store in fridge for up to a week.
OR
6. Pour broth into muffin tins and freeze, then bag for later use.

PRESSURE COOKER DIRECTIONS:

1. Chop vegetables into large chunks.
2. Place all ingredients in a pressure cooker.
3. Cook on high presssure for 1 hour.
4. Strain mixture through a dishtowel-lined colander.
5. Pour broth into mason jars and store in fridge for up to a week.
OR
6. Pour broth into muffin tins and freeze, then bag for later use.

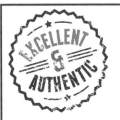

3 HOMEMADE SEASONING MIXES

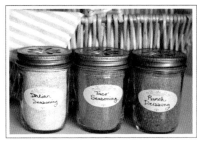

ITALIAN SEASONING:
- 2 TBS. garlic powder
- 4 TBS. onion powder
- 2 1/2 TBS. dried oregano
- 4 TBS. dried parsley
- 2 1/2 TBS. salt
- 1 TBS. pepper
- 1 tsp. dried thyme
- 2 tsp. celery flakes

1. Mix all ingredients in a food processor and blend. Store in a jar.

For Italian Dressing:
Mix 2 TBS. Homemade Mix with 1/4 c. apple cider vinegar, 1 TBS. water, & 1/2 c. olive oil.

TACO SEASONING:
- 1/3 c. chili powder
- 3 TBS. onion powder
- 1 1/2 TBS. cumin
- 1 TBS. garlic powder
- 1 TBS. paprika
- 1 TBS. salt

1. Mix all ingredients. Store in a jar.

For Tacos:
Mix 3 TBS. of Homemade Mix with 2 TBS. of arrowroot powder & 3 TBS. water to 1 lb. of ground beef

RANCH DRESSING:
- 1/2 c. dried chives
- 3/4 c. parsley
- 2 TBS. garlic powder
- 2 tsp. paprika

1. Mix all ingredients in a food processor and blend. Store in jar.

For Ranch Dressing:
Mix 1 TBS. of Homemade Mix with 1/2 c. of organic mayo, 1 c. of whole milk yogurt, & 1 tsp. of honey.

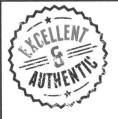

FRESH & EASY SALSA

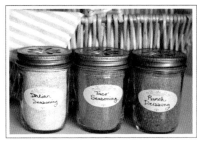

INGREDIENTS:
- 4 ripe tomatoes or a BPA-free can of diced tomatoes
- 1 handful of fresh cilantro
- 2 diced garlic cloves or 1/2 tsp. of garlic powder
- 1 TBS. of raw honey
- 1 squeeze of lime
- 1 can of diced green chilies
- 1/2 medium sweet vidalia onion, diced.
- salt & pepper to taste

DIRECTIONS:
1. Combine all ingredients in a blender and pulse till desired consistency is reached.

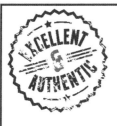

HOMEMADE BBQ SAUCE

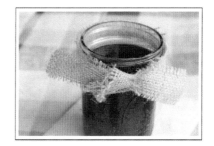

INGREDIENTS:

- 2 TBS. lard, tallow, or coconut oil
- 1/4 c. water
- 6 oz. tomato paste
- 1/4 c. apple cider vinegar
- 2 TBS. molasses
- 1/2 c. maple syrup or honey
- 1 1/2 TBS. onion powder
- 1/2 TBS. garlic powder
- 1/2 tsp. chili powder
- 1/8 tsp. cayenne pepper
- 3/4 tsp. salt
- 1/2 tsp. natural liquid smoke
- 2 TBS. pureed raw liver (optional)

DIRECTIONS:

1. Mix all ingredients in a saucepan over medium-high heat.
2. While stirring, bring to a boil, then remove from heat and let cool.

TIP- Store in the fridge for up to 3 months (only 1 month if you added liver), or freezer for up to 6 months.

YIELDS 2 CUPS

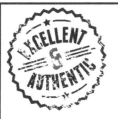

HOMEMADE ENCHILADA SAUCE

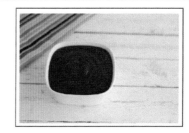

INGREDIENTS:

- 1/4 c. tallow, lard, or coconut oil
- 1 can or jar of organic tomato sauce
- 1/4 c. chili powder
- 1/4 tsp. cumin
- 1/4 tsp. garlic powder
- 1/4 tsp. onion powder
- 2 TBS. organic corn starch or arrowroot starch
- 1 1/2 c. filtered water

DIRECTIONS:

1. Mix all ingredients in a saucepan and bring to a boil.
2. Remove from heat and let cool.

YIELD 1 QUART

BREADS

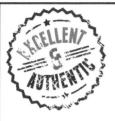

HOMEMADE SOAKED
TORTILLAS

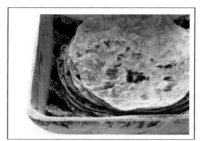

INGREDIENTS:

- 2 c. whole-wheat flour
- 1/4 c. lard, tallow, or coconut oil
- 3/4 c. filtered water + 1-2 tablespoons if it seems dry.
- 1 TBS. acidic medium (apple cider vinegar, whey, yogurt, kefir)

- 1 tsp. salt
arrowroot powder for rolling

DIRECTIONS:

1. Mix flour & lard together with a pastry cutter.
2. Add water & acidic medium, then mix together well with spoon. Make sure all flour is wet. Let sit at room temperature for 12 hours.
3. Add salt and mix into dough with hands. Let rest for 5 min.
4. Heat a skillet over medium-high heat.
5. Divide dough into 8 sections.
6. Roll out a tortilla on arrowroot powder dusted counter top, then cook on ungreased skillet for about 30 seconds on each side. Best if cooked slightly underdone. Repeat for remaining tortillas.

MAKES 8 TORTILLAS

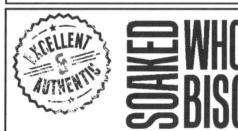

SOAKED WHOLE-GRAIN
BISCUITS

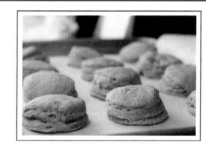

INGREDIENTS:

- 2 c. whole-wheat flour
- 1/3 c. lard, tallow, coconut oil, or butter
- 1 c. milk – we drink raw milk, read why here.
- 2 TBS. apple cider vinegar

- 3 tsp. baking powder
- 1/4 tsp. baking soda
- 1/2 tsp. of salt

- A couple tablespoons of arrowroot powder or organic cornstarch for rolling out dough

DIRECTIONS:

1. Using a pastry cutter, cut lard into flour until the mixture resembles tiny grains.
2. Add 2 Tbs. of apple cider vinegar to 1 c. of milk.
3. Make a well in the flour mixture, then pour the liquid mixture into the middle, mixing well.
4. Cover the bowl with saran wrap and let sit on your counter for 12-24 hours. I usually just soak mine overnight.
5. After 12-24 hours, remove saran wrap and add baking powder, baking soda, & salt.
6. Mix by folding dough over itself about 6-8 times. Be careful not to over mix.
7. Dust a counter top with some arrowroot powder, then roll out dough with a rolling pin to about 1/2 inch thickness.
Cut into circle-shaped biscuits, and place on a baking sheet lined with parchment paper.
8. Bake at 350 degrees for 12-18 minutes, or until slightly brown.

SERVES 6-8

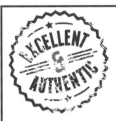

SOAKED CORNBREAD

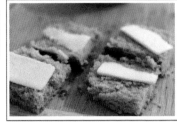

INGREDIENTS:

- 2 c. cornmeal
- 1 c. whole-wheat flour + 1 c. organic white flour
(or 2 c. of whole wheat flour is fine, too.)
- 2 c. milk
- 2 TBS. apple cider vinegar
----

4 eggs
1 stick of melted butter
2 tsp. salt
1 tsp. baking soda
2 TBS. baking powder
4 TBS. unrefined cane sugar or coconut sugar

DIRECTIONS:

1. In a bowl, place 2 c. of cornmeal & flour. Mix together milk & apple cider vinegar, then add to cornmeal/flour mixture.
2. Mix until just combined, then cover with plastic wrap nice and tight, and let sit on your counter top at room temperature for 8-12 hours.
3. After 8-12 hours, add rest of ingredients but be sure not to overmix.
4. Place in a 9×13 greased pan and bake at 375 degrees for 35-40 minutes, or when a toothpick inserted comes out clean.
(TIP – If it starts to look too brown, you can cover it with some aluminum foil for the last 10 min. or so)

SERVES 6-8

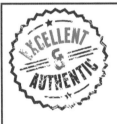

HOMEMADE SOAKED BREAD

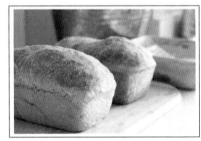

INGREDIENTS:

- 3 c. water
- 2 TBS. of an acidic medium (apple cider vinegar, whey, yogurt, kefir)
- 7 1/2 c. of whole-wheat flour

- 1/4 c. water
- 2 TBS. unrefined cane sugar or coconut sugar
- 2 heaping tsp. of active dry yeast (not instant)

- 2 tsp. salt
- 1/2 crushed tablet of Vitamin C (ascorbic acid)

arrowroot powder for dusting countertop

DIRECTIONS:

1. Mix flour, water, & acidic medium until well incorporated. Cover with a greased plastic wrap and sit at room temperature for 12-24 hours.
2. After 12-24 hours, warm dough for 10 minutes by placing in a warm oven.
3. Mix warm water, yeast, & sweetener and add to dough. Mix well by kneading with hands. Cover with greased plastic wrap and let rise in a warm oven for 30-45 minutes or until doubled.
4. After 30-45 minutes, sprinkle 2 tsp. of salt & 1/2 crushed tablet of Vitamin C (ascorbic acid) and knead well with hands until the dough is tough and the gluten is well formed. Divide dough in half and flatten out each peice into a rectabgle on counter top that is dusted with arrowroot starch. Roll each loaf and tuck the ends. Butter two bread pans and place each loaf in it's pan. Place in a warm oven & let rise, uncovered, another 30-45 minutes.
5. After 30-45 minutes, carefully remove risen bread out of oven and preheat the oven to 350 degrees.
6. Bake the bread at 350 degrees for 40 minutes or until internal temp. reaches 180 degrees. Remove bread and let cool in pans for 5 minutes, then remove & let cool for 10-25 minutes before cutting.

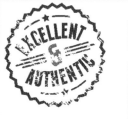

QUIICK ROLLS

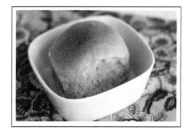

INGREDIENTS:

- 2 c. filtered water
- 3 TBS. butter
- 3 TBS. honey
- 1 1/2 tsp. salt
- 3 c. sprouted flour
- 2 tsp. active dry yeast
- 2 c. white flour

DIRECTIONS:

1. Mix all ingredients.
2. Knead for 6 minutes with either a dough hook in a mixer or by hand.
3. Place dough in a bowl, cover with cloth and place in a warm spot for 30 minutes.
4. Form into rolls and place in a greased pan.
5. Let rise 20-30 minutes in a warm spot or until doubled in size.
6. Bake at 350 for 20 minutes or until internal temperature reaches 180 degrees.

NOTE* You can preheat the oven to 350 for 1 minute, then turn it off to create a warm spot for your rising periods.

YIELDS 24 ROLLS

FERMENTED FOODS

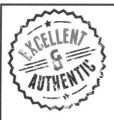

HOMEMADE
SODA aka WATER KEFIR

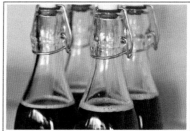

JUICE METHOD:

- 1/4 c. water kefir grains
- 3-5 mineral drops
- 1/2 gallon of Organic juice, fresh or storebought

----

1. Add water kefir grains to juice. Cover loosely with cloth & leave on counter at room temperature for 12 hours.
2. Pour soda into bottles or one big jar and cover tightly with a lid. Leave on counter another 12 hours.
3. Refridgerate and enjoy the fizziness!

WATER METHOD:

- 1/4 c. water kefir grains
- 3-5 mineral drops
- 1/2 gallon of filtered water
- 1/2 c. organic cane sugar
- 1 c. low acidic juice (apple, grape, cherry) or 1 peel from an ORGANIC acidic fruit (lemon, lime, orange, grapefruit)

----

1. Mix water kefir grain, minerals, water, & sugar. Cover loosely with cloth & leave on counter at room temperature for 12 hours.
2. Pour soda into bottles or one big jar, add juice or peel and cover tightly with a lid. Leave on counter another 12 hours.
3. Refrigerate and enjoy the fizziness!

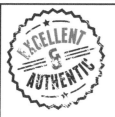

HOMEMADE
YOGURT

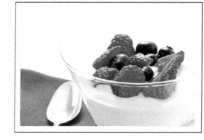

INGREDIENTS:

- 1 quart whole milk
- 1/8 tsp. of freeze-dried starter culture OR 2 TBS. of yogurt from a previous batch.

DIRECTIONS:

1. Heat milk in saucepan, stirring constantly, until the temperature reaches 180F degrees. (This is not to pasteurize it, but to breakdown the protein molecules so your yogurt will be thicker)
2. Cool milk to 115 degrees, then add yogurt culture)
3. Stir well and pour into either a yogurt maker or crockpot insulated in a cooler and let it sit undisturbed at 105-110F for 7-8 hours.
4. Refrigerate to solidify, then enjoy!

BREAKFAST

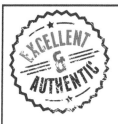

SPROUTED WHEAT PANCAKES

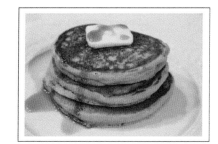

INGREDIENTS:

- 2 c. sprouted wheat flour
- 2 eggs
- 2 c. whole milk
- 1 heaping tsp. sea salt
- 1 heaping TBS. baking powder
- 1-3 TBS. coconut oil, for cooking.

DIRECTIONS:

1. Mix flour, eggs, milk, salt, & baking powder.
2. Pour onto hot greased griddle and cook about 2-3 minutes on each side.

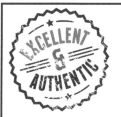

OVERNIGHT-SOAKED OATMEAL

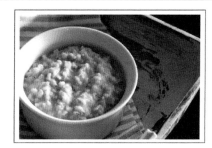

INGREDIENTS:

- 4 c. filtered water
- 2 c. rolled oats
- 1 TBS. acidic medium of your choice (apple cider vinegar, yogurt, kefir, whey)
- 1/2 tsp. salt

TOPPINGS:
- butter
- milk or cream
- nuts
- fruit
- maple syrup, honey, etc.

SERVES 6-8

DIRECTIONS:

1. Place water, oats, & acidic medium in a saucepan. Leave on your countertop overnight. (10-12 hours)
2. In the morning, add salt and bring to a boil, then remove from heat and let sit covered for 10 minutes.
3. Serve with as many toppings as you want!

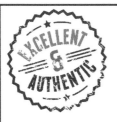

THE BEST SCRAMBLED EGGS

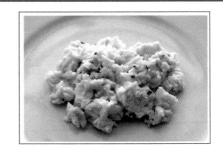

INGREDIENTS:

- 8 eggs
- 2 TBS. cream
- 1 TBS. fresh chopped chives
- 1 tsp. butter

DIRECTIONS:

1. Heat pan over medium-high heat and grease with butter.
2. In a bowl, whisk eggs, cream & chives.
3. Pour egg mixture in pan and stir while cooking until almost completely cooked, but remove while still a bit wet.
4. Serve warm & enjoy!

SERVES 6-8

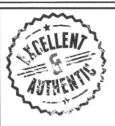

SOAKED GRANOLA

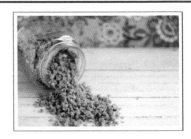

INGREDIENTS:

- 1 c. of butter or coconut oil
- 1 can of coconut milk
- 2 c. of filtered water
- 4 TBS. of acidic medium
- 6 c. rolled oats

- 1 c. honey or maple syrup
- 1 tsp. sea salt
- 1 tsp. vanilla
- 1 TBS. ground cinnamon

DIRECTIONS:

1. Mix butter, coconut milk, water, & acidic medium in a saucepan over low heat.
2. Once your ingredients are melted and well mixed, pour over rolled oats and soak, covered, for 12-24 hours.
3. After your oats have soaked for 12-24 hours, mix honey, salt, vanilla, & cinnamon in a bowl and add to oats.
4. Mix well, then spread out on two parchment paper-lined baking sheets and bake at 170 degrees for 4-6 hours, turning and breaking up the granola every 2 hours.
5. Remove when slightly brown and still slightly moist.
6. Allow to cool and air dry, then store in an airtight container for up to 2 weeks.

YIELD 6 CUPS

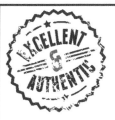

SPROUTED FLOUR WAFFLES

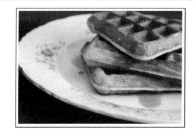

INGREDIENTS:

Ingredients:
- 2 c. sprouted wheat flour
- 2 eggs
- 2 c. milk
- 2 TBS. coconut oil or pastured lard
- 1 heaping tsp. sea salt
- 1 heaping TBS. baking powder

DIRECTIONS:

1. Preheat a waffle-maker.
2. Mix all ingredients and pour into waffle-maker.
3. Top with real butter & maple syrup and enjoy!

SERVES 6-8

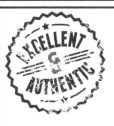

WHOLE-GRAIN CREPES

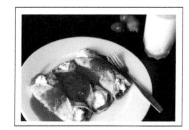

INGREDIENTS:

Crepe Ingredients:
3 eggs
1 c. sprouted flour
1 1/4 c. milk
1 TBS. honey
1 tsp. vanilla
1/4 tsp. salt
2 TBS. coconut oil for greasing skillet

Berry Sauce Ingredients:
1 c. any kind of berries
1 TBS. water

Whipped Cream Ingredients:
1 c. whole cream
1 TBS. unrefined sugar

DIRECTIONS:

1. Mix all crepe ingredients in blender and puree. Place blender pitcher in fridge for 15 mintues.
2. In a small saucepan over medium heat, mix berries and water. Allow to cook 5 mintues, then remove from heat and set aside.
3. In a small bowl, whip the cream at high speed with a hand mixer. Once the cream starts to thicken, add sugar and stop blending once whipped cream forms.
4. Heat a small pan over medium heat and grease with coconut oil.
5. Pour just enough crepe batter to cover the bottom of the pan. Cook for 1-2 minutes on each side and use a thin spatula to flip.
6. Continue cooking crepes until the batter is gone.
7. Clean out blender and puree cooked berries.
8. Serve crepes with fruit, whipped cream, & berry sauce.

SERVES 6-8

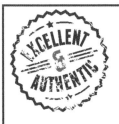

SWEET POTATO
HASH

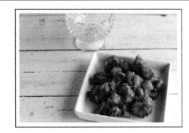

INGREDIENTS:

- 4-5 leftover baked sweet potatoes
- 6 TBS. tallow, lard, or coconut oil
- salt n' pepper

DIRECTIONS:

1. Peel & dice leftover sweet potatoes.
2. Heat oil in frying pan over medium-high heat.
3. Saute potatoes in oil until browned.
4. Remove from heat, top with salt and pepper to taste, and serve!

SERVES 6-8

LUNCHES

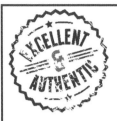

GRILLED CHEESE SANDWICHES

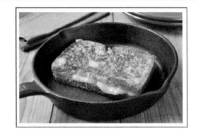

INGREDIENTS:

Ingredients:
- 12 slices bread
- 1 stick butter, room temperature
- 6 slices of real cheddar cheese

DIRECTIONS:

1. Preheat a skillet to medium heat.
2. Butter one side of each piece of bread.
3. Place bread in skillet butter side up. Once the butter has melted, flip over and add cheddar cheese to the toasted un-buttered side.
4. Place one piece of bread on another to form a sandwich. Make sure both sides are toasted evenly and the cheese is melted. Be careful not to burn the bread.

SERVES 6

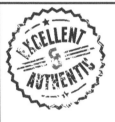

EGG SALAD

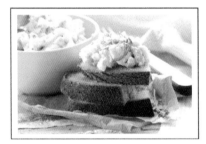

INGREDIENTS:

- 6 hard boiled eggs
- 4 TBS. organic mayo
- 2 tsp. mustard
- salt n' pepper

DIRECTIONS:

1. Mix all ingredients and eat on bread or in a lettuce wrap.

SERVES 6-8

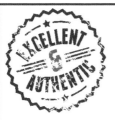

TUNA SALAD

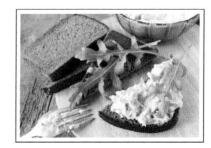

INGREDIENTS:

- 2 can wild-caught albacore tuna
- 4 TBS. organic mayo
- 2 tsp. mustard
- 1 celery sticks, minced
- salt n' pepper

DIRECTIONS:

1. 1. Mix all ingredients and eat on bread or in a lettuce wrap.

SERVES 6-8

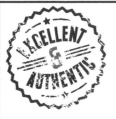

CHICKEN SALAD

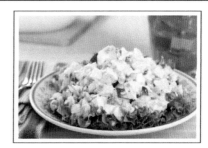

INGREDIENTS:

- 2 c. cooked, shredded chicken or 2 cans of organic, canned chicken
- 3 TBS. mayo
- 1 TBS. yogurt
- 2 celery sticks, diced
- 1 c. grapes, sliced into halves
- 2 green onions, diced
- 1 apple, diced
- 1/2 c. pecans or walnuts, diced
- salt n' pepper

DIRECTIONS:

1. Mix all ingredients and eat on bread or in a lettuce wrap.

SERVES 6-8

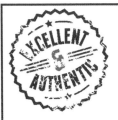

WALDORF SALAD

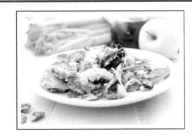

INGREDIENTS:
- 2 lbs. mixed greens
- 4 apples
- 1/2 bunch grapes
- 6 oz. blue cheese
- 2 c. pecans
- 2 TBS. butter
- 1 TBS. unrefined sugar
salt n' pepper

For dressing:
olive oil
balsamic vinegar

DIRECTIONS:
1. In a pan over medium-high heat, melt butter & sugar. Add pecans and cook for 2-3 minutes.
2. Arrange salad with rest of ingredients, and pour olive oil & balsamic vinegar over the top. Enjoy!

NOTE* for added digestibility, soak nuts for 4-8 hours prior to cooking.

SERVES 6-8

SNACKS

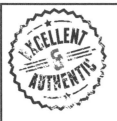

CREAM CHEESE & APPLE SANDWICHES

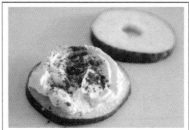

INGREDIENTS:

- 3 apples
- 8 oz. full-fat cream cheese
- 1 tsp. cinnamon

DIRECTIONS:

1. Wash and slice apples horizontally to make circles.
2. Cut out middle core of each circle.
3. On one slice of apple, spread cream cheese, sprinkle cinnamon, and top with another slice of apple.
4. Enjoy!

SERVES 6-8

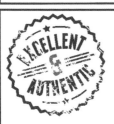

FUDGE-SICLES

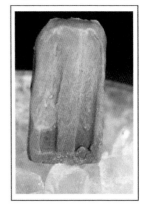

INGREDIENTS:

- 3 bananas
- 1 can coconut milk
- 2 cups of water
- 1 tsp. vanilla
- 3 TBS. cocoa
- pinch of salt

DIRECTIONS:

1. Mix all ingredients in your blender.
2. Pour into popsicle molds and freeze for at least 4-5 hours.

SERVES 6-8

DINNERS

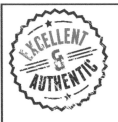

HEARTY & MOIST
MEATLOAF

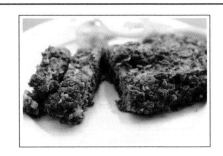

INGREDIENTS:

- 1 lb. hamburger
- 1 egg
- 1 can BPA-free tomato sauce (or 4 crushed tomatoes)
- 1/2 c. grated carrots
- 1/4 c. diced celery
- 1/4 medium onion, minced
- 1/4 c. rolled oats or bread crumbs
- 1/8 tsp. garlic
- 1/2 tsp. salt
- 1/4 tsp. pepper

DIRECTIONS:

1. Mix all ingredients in a bowl, but don't overmix.
2. Form 2 loafs, each about 2 inches high in baking dish.
3. Bake at 350 degrees for 30-40 minutes, or until top is well-browned

SERVES 6-8

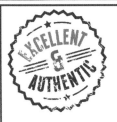

MANGO-QUINOA
SALAD

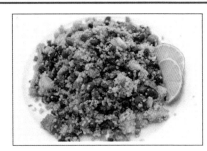

INGREDIENTS:

- 2 c. cooked quinoa
- 1 1/2 c. black beans, cooked & drained
- 2 medium mangos, peeled & diced
- 1 red bell pepper, diced
- 6 green onions, thinly sliced
- 1 handful chopped cilantro (about 1/2 cup)

Dressing
- 2 TBS. apple cider vinegar
- 4 TBS. olive oil
- 2 TBS. fresh lime juice
- 2 TBS. honey
- salt & pepper to taste

DIRECTIONS:

1. Place cooked quinoa in a large bowl.
2. Add mango, red pepper, green onion, black beans, and cilantro.
3. In a small bowl, combine vinegar, olive oil, lime juice, & honey.
4. Whisk until smooth and pour over top of salad.
5. Toss to combine and add salt & pepper to taste.
6. Chill & serve.

SERVES 6-8

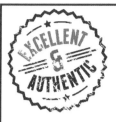

CRISPY SALMON
PATTIES

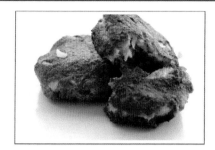

INGREDIENTS:

- 2 can wild salmon, drained
- 3 eggs
- 1/2 c. seasoned dry bread crumbs
- 1/2 c. dry potato flakes
- 1/2 medium onion
- 1 clove garlic, minced
- 1 tsp. dried dill weed
- 1 tsp. celery salt
- 1/2 c. coconut oil, lard, or tallow

DIRECTIONS:

1. In a medium bowl, mix all ingredients except coconut oil.
2. In a frying pan, heat coconut oil on medium-high heat and fry the salmon patties about 3 minutes on each side, until golden brown.
3. Serve with a side of rice or salad or as an appetizer.

SERVES 6-8

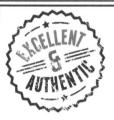

SWEET N' SOUR
CHICKEN

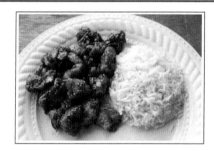

INGREDIENTS:

- 2 lbs. Organic chicken tenders or thighs
- 3/4 c. arrowroot starch
- 2 pasture-raised eggs
- 1/4 c. coconut oil

Sauce:
- 1/2 c. honey or cane sugar
- 4 TBS. Organic ketchup
- 1/2 c. apple cider vinegar
- 1 TBS. organic or fermented soy sauce
- 1 tsp. garlic powder

DIRECTIONS:

1. Dice chicken into 1-inch pieces.
2. Place in a bowl, coat with arrowroot starch.
3. Whisk eggs in another bowl. Dip coated chicken in eggs.
4. Heat coconut oil in a pan over medium-high heat.
5. Fry chicken until golden brown.
6. In separate bowl, mix sauce ingredients thoroughly.
7. Place chicken in baking dish and pour sauce over it. Bake at 325 degrees for 30 minutes, stirring every 10 minutes.
8. Serve with a side of organic white rice, wild rice, or brown rice.

SERVES 6-8

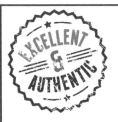

ASIAN VEGGIE STIR-FRY

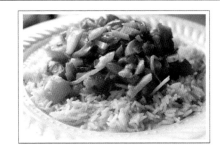

INGREDIENTS:

- 2 TBS. coconut oil, lard, or tallow
- 2 peppers, any color
- 1/2 onion
- 1 c. bean sprouts
- 1 c. mushrooms
- 1 c. diced zucchini
- 1 can of water chestnuts
- salt n' pepper to taste

Sauce:
- 1 TBS. butter
- 1 TBS. organic or fermented soy sauce
- 1 TBS. arrowroot powder
- 1 c. homemade broth

SERVES 6-8

DIRECTIONS:

1. Melt oil in large frying pan over medium-high heat.
2. Place all veggies in the pan and saute about 15 minutes.
3. Mix sauce ingredients together and pour over veggies and cook an additional 5 minutes.
4. Serve over organic white rice, wild rice, or brown rice.

NAVAJO TACOS

SERVES 6-8

DOUGH INGREDIENTS:

- 4 1/2 c. whole-wheat or spelt flour
- 2 1/4 c. warm water
- 2 TBS. acidic medium (apple cider vinegar, whey, yogurt, kefir, or lemon juice)

- 1 3/4 tsp. sea salt
- 2 heaping tsp. active dry yeast
- 1 TBS. melted butter
- 1 TBS. honey
- 1/2 c. arrowroot powder, divided
- 1 c. coconut oil (for pan frying_

BEANS INGREDIENTS:

- 2 c. pinto beans
- 1 TBS. acidic medium of your choice

DOUGH DIRECTIONS:

1. Combine flour, water, & 2 TBS. of acidic medium in a bowl. Mix with a spoon until well incorporated and wet.
2. Cover with a greased saran wrap and a twole tightly so it won't dry out. Leave at room temperature for 12 hours.
4. After 12 hours, add yeast, butter, honey, & salt & mix well in bowl.
5. Cover again and let rise for 30 minutes.
6. Heat oil in pan over med-high heat. Sprinkle arrowroot powder on dough and on countertop. Grab a golf-ball sized peice of dough and form to a 5 inch circle. Fry those puppies up about 1 min. on each side.

BEANS INGREDIENTS:

1. Place 2 c. of beans in a big bowl. Cover completely with water and 1 TBS. of acidic medium. Soak 8-12 hours.
2. After 8-12 hours, cook either in a pressure cooker on high for 30 min. or on the stove top for 4 hours. Drain & mash beans & add salt.
TOPPINGS: cheese, avocado, lettuce, tomato, cilantro

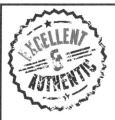

THE ULTIMATE
BAKED POTATO

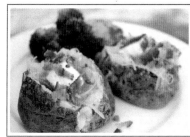

INGREDIENTS:

- 8-10 large potatoes, scrubbed clean
- 1/2 c. coconut oil
- 2 tsp. sea salt

Toppings:
- butter
- cheese
- sour cream
- bacon
- steamed broccoli

OVEN DIRECTIONS:

1. Wash potatoes & prick with a fork a couple times.
2. Place potatoes on a baking sheet.
3. Drizzle coconut oil and sea salt over the top.
4. Bake at 350 degrees for 60 minutes.
5. Top with toppings.

CROCKPOT DIRECTIONS:

1. Wash potatoes & prick with a fork a couple times.
2. Drizzle coconut oil and salt over potatoes, then wrap each potato individually in aluminum foil.
3. Place in crockpot and cook on LOW for 8-10 hours.

SERVES 6-8

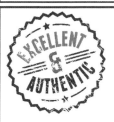

LIGHT & FLUFFY
PIZZA

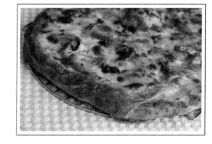

INGREDIENTS:

- 4 1/2 c. whole-wheat flour
- 2 1/4 c. warm water
- 2 TBS. acidic medium (apple cider vinegar, whey, yogurt, kefir, or lemon juice)
- 1 3/4 tsp. sea salt

- 2 heaping tsp. dry yeast
- 1 TBS. honey
- 2 TBS. olive oil
- 1/2 c. arrowroot powder, divided
- 1 c. coconut oil (for pan frying)

DIRECTIONS:

1. Combine flour, water, 2 TBS. of acidic medium, and salt in a bowl. Mix with a spoon until well incorporated and wet.
2. Cover with a greased saran wrap and a towel tightly so it won't dry out. Leave at room temperature for 12 hours.
----
4. After 12 hours, add yeast, and honey & mix well in bowl.
5. . Divide the dough into 2 sections for 2 deep dish pizzas or 3 sections for 3 thin crust pizzas
6. Pour olive oil in separate bowls & place dough in separate bowls on top of oil, and cover again and let rise for 30 minutes.
7. Preheat oven with pizza stone inside to 500F degrees
8. Sprinkle arrowroot powder on dough and on parchment paper.
9. To roll out, dump contents of one bowl onto parchment paper. Lightly press out with fingers, keeping bubbles intact. Top with toppings and bake for 8-10 minutes with paper directly on pizza stone at 500F degrees
10. Remove by sliding cutting board under paper, let cool & slice.

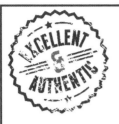

ASIAN LETTUCE
WRAPS

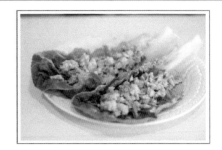

INGREDIENTS:

- 2 lb. ground chicken
- 1 c. cashews, chopped
- 2 can water chestnuts, chopped
- 1/2 medium onion, chopped
- 1 clove garlic, minced
- 1 inch knob of fresh ginger, grated
SAUCE:
- 2 TBS. sesame oil
- 5 TBS. Coconut Aminos (soy sauce)
- 2 TBS. peanut butter (or any other nut butter)
- 3 TBS. honey
- 2 TBS. red wine or rice vinegar
- 1/2 tsp. chili powder

- One head of romaine or iceburg lettuce

DIRECTIONS:

1. Saute onion in a little oil. Add chicken, and cook until no longer pink. Add cashews, water chestnuts, garlic, & ginger. Reduce heat to simmer.
2. Mix all sauce ingredients in saucepan. Heat until combined. Add to chicken mixture and simmer until sauce is thickened. Serve hot or cold with freshly washed lettuce.

SERVES 6-8

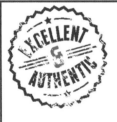

CHICKEN ENCHILADAS

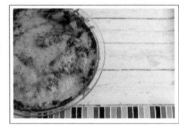

INGREDIENTS:

- 1 quart of Homemade Enchilada Sauce
- 3 c. cheddar cheese
- 1 pkg. of organic sprouted corn tortillas
- 2 c. shredded, cooked chicken

DIRECTIONS:

1. In a glass casserole dish, layer sauce, tortillas, chicken, cheese.
2. Repeat.
3. Top with cheese and bake at 350 for 30 minutes.

SERVES 6-8

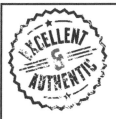

FAJITAS

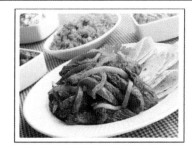

INGREDIENTS:

- 1 medium onion, sliced
- 2 peppers (any color), sliced
- 2 TBS. tallow, lard, or coconut oil
- 1 lb. meat (steak, chicken, lamb)
- 1 pkg. Organic Sprouted Corn Tortillas

Toppings:
sour cream
avocados

DIRECTIONS:

1. Saute onion & peppers in oil in a pan over medium heat.
2. Add meat and cook until browned.
3. Remove onion, peppers, & meat from pan.
4. Lightly cook tortillas in oil until warm.
5. Serve with toppings.

SERVES 6-8

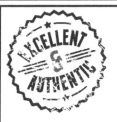

HONEY GLAZED SALMON

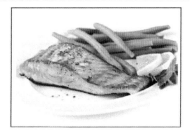

INGREDIENTS:

Ingredients:
- 6 pieces of wild-caught salmon
- 3 TBS. olive oil
- 1 TBS. honey
- 1/2 tsp. garlic powder
- salt n' pepper

DIRECTIONS:

1. Preheat oven to 350 degrees.
2. In a small bowl, mix olive oil, honey, & garlic powder.
3. Place salmon in a glass baking dish and pour glaze over salmon.
4. Bake for 12-15 minutes.

SERVES 6-8

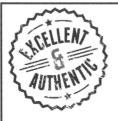

CROCKPOT 3-CHEESE VEGGIE LASAGNA

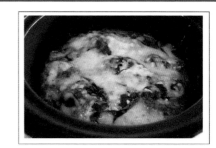

INGREDIENTS:

- 2 cans BPA-free organic tomato sauce
(or 10 tomatoes, crushed)
- 4 TBS. homemade dry italian seasoning
- 2 TBS. olive oil
- 2 TBS. honey or cane sugar
- 1/2 c. water
- 16 oz. whole-fat cottage cheese
- 2 cups whole-fat mozzarella cheese
- 1 cup parmesean cheese
- 2 eggs
- 1/2 tsp. salt
- 1/4 tsp. pepper
- 2 medium sized zucchinis
- 2 cups fresh mushrooms
- 3 cups fresh spinach
- (optional) 1 pkg. whole grain pasta

DIRECTIONS:

1. In a small bowl, combine tomato sauce with italian seasoning, olive oil, & sweetener.
2. In another bowl, combine water, cottage cheese, 2 eggs, salt, & pepper.
3. Slice zucchinis and wash mushrooms & spinach.
4. Place some sauce on the bottom, then layer the in the crockpot as follows: veggies and/or noodles, cottage cheese/egg mixture, mozzarella cheese. Repeat.
5. Top with parmesan cheese.

6. Cook on low for 4 hours or high for 2 hours.

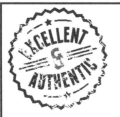

MAC N' CHEESE

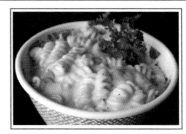

INGREDIENTS:

- 16 oz. pasta (my latest favorite is Einkorn pasta)
- 8 TBS. butter
- 4 TBS. organic corn starch
- 3 c. whole milk
- 3-4 c. shredded cheddar cheese
- salt & pepper to taste

DIRECTIONS:

1. Cook pasta according to instructions.
2. In a pot over medium heat, melt butter, then add corn starch and stir well.
3. Add milk and bring to a simmer while stirring constantly.
4. Add shredded cheese and stir until the cheese is melted and the sauce has thickened.
5. Remove from heat and add to cooked pasta, then add salt and pepper to your taste.

SERVES 6-8

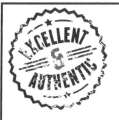

ULTIMATE NACHOS

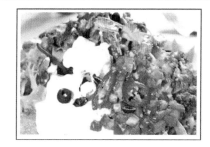

INGREDIENTS:

- 2 large bags of Organic Corn Chips
- 4 c. cheddar cheese
- 1 lb. ground beef
- 3 TBS. Homemade Taco Seasoning
- 2 TBS. organic corn starch or arrowroot starch
- 3 TBS. filtered water

Toppings:
sour cream, tomatoes, olives, salsa, guacamole

DIRECTIONS:

1. In a pan over medium heat, brown ground beef.
2. Add Homemade Taco Seasoning, starch, & water.
3. Cook an additional 2 minutes, then remove from heat.
4. On a big baking sheet, lay out chips, cheese, & ground beef.
5. Warm in oven until cheese is melted, then remove from oven and top with toppings!

SERVES 6-8

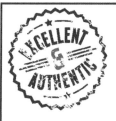

SLOW-COOKER POT ROAST

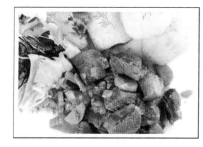

INGREDIENTS:

- 5 lb. rump roast
- 1/2 medium onion
- 1 lb. carrots, cut into 3 inch pieces
- 6 red or russet potatoes, quartered
- 1 sprig of rosemary & thyme
- 2 c. filtered water

DIRECTIONS:

1. Heat a pan over high heat.
2. Salt & pepper the roast, then brown on all sides.
3. Place roast in crockpot, then add onion, carrots, potatoes, water, rosemary, & thyme.
4. Cook on high for 4 hours or low for 6-8 hours.

SERVES 6-8

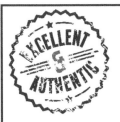

ROAST CHICKEN

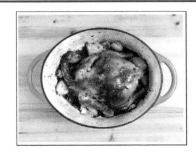

INGREDIENTS:

- 1 whole chicken
- 1 stick butter, cubed.
- 1/2 medium onion
- 1 lemon, quartered.
- 2 garlic cloves
- 1/2 tsp. thyme
- 1/2 tsp. oregano
- salt n' pepper

DIRECTIONS:

1. Generously salt and pepper the inside cavity of the chicken, and stuff with garlic cloves, onion, 1/2 of the butter, & lemon.
2. Put the other half of the butter under the skin of the chicken, and sprinkle the outside of the chicken with thyme, oregano, & more salt & pepper.
3. Place in a roasting dish cover and bake at 375 for 1 hour. (Place any root vegetables around the sides if you want)
4. Remove cover and bake 1 hour. (if it starts to get too brown, cover for the rest of baking time)
5. Let cool 10-15 minutes before cutting.

SERVES 6-8

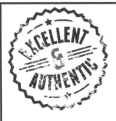

PERFECT GRILLED STEAK

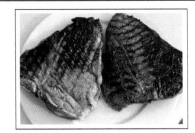

INGREDIENTS:

CHOOSE A STEAK:
- Porterhouse
- Rib-eye
- T-bone
- Top Sirloin
- NY Strip, or any other kind of steak with the word "strip" in it.

Ingredients:
- 6-8 steaks
- salt n' pepper

DIRECTIONS:

1. Start by gettin' your grill pan screamin' hot.
2. Throw some pats of butter on your grill and let it melt.
3. Lay your seasoned steaks on your grill and be sure not to move it around until a minute passes.
4. After a minute, rotate them a bit to create some cool looking criss cross action. Let it cook for another minute.
5. Now flip 'em over and do the same thing on the other side. After each side has been seared, lower the heat down to medium and just let them hang out until your desired cooking length.

SERVES 6-8

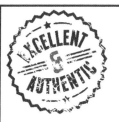

BEAN & CHEESE
TOSTADAS

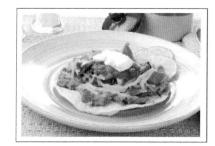

INGREDIENTS:

- 2 c. beans
- 1 TBS. apple cider vinegar

- 1 pkg. Organic Sprouted Corn Tortillas
- 1/2 c. tallow, lard, or coconut oil

Toppings:
lettuce, cheese, tomatoes, avocados, cilantro

DIRECTIONS:

BEANS Directions:
1. Place beans in a big bowl. Cover completely with water and 1 TBS. of apple cider vinegar.
2. Soak 8-12 hours.
3. After 8-12 hours cook either in a pressure cooker on high for 30 minutes or in a crockpot on low for 6-8 hours.
4. Drain, mash beans & add salt.

TORTILLAS Directions:
1. Heat oil in a small saucepan to 375 degrees.
2. Fry tortillas one at a time until crispy & lightly browned.

SERVES 6-8

SOUPS

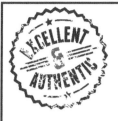

BUTTERNUT SQUASH
SOUP

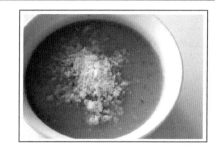

INGREDIENTS:

- 2 medium butternut squash
- 1/2 onion, diced
- 1 clove garlic, minced
- 4 TBS. olive oil, tallow, lard, or butter
- 1/4 tsp. chili powder
- a pinch of nutmeg
- 4 c. chicken broth
- 1 tsp. salt
- 1/2 tsp. pepper
TOP with freshly grated parmesan cheese

DIRECTIONS:

1. Cut each squash into 2-3 pieces, but don't peel. Be careful, these buggers are hard to cut! Cook either in a pressure cooker for 5 minutes on high pressure, or steam on the stove top about 30 minutes.
2. In a pan over medium heat, saute onion & garlic in oil 5-7 minutes or until translucent.
3. Remove peel from squash, then puree all ingredients in a blender until desired consistency is reached.
4. Top with parmesan cheese & enjoy!

SERVES 6-8

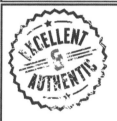

CHEESY BROCCOLI
SOUP

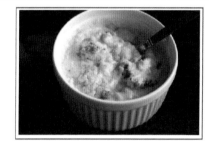

INGREDIENTS:

- 8 large potatoes, diced
- 1 onion, diced
- 4 TBS. olive oil, tallow, lard, or butter
- 4 c. chicken broth
- 6 c. cheddar cheese (about 1.5 lbs)
- 2 c. sour cream
- 2 head of broccoli
- 1/2 tsp. salt
- 1/2 tsp. pepper

DIRECTIONS:

1. Dice potatoes, then add to a pot of boiling salted water. Cook for 10-12 minutes or until tender.
2. In a large pot over medium heat, saute onion in oil.
3. When potatoes are tender, drain & then add to sauteed onions.
4. Add chicken broth & broccoli and cook until broccoli is tender (about 7-10 minutes), then add cheese & sour cream & cook until well mixed.
5. Remove from heat and devour!

SERVES 6-8

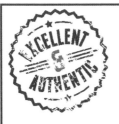

CHICKEN NOODLE SOUP

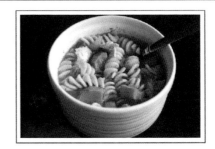

INGREDIENTS:

- 16 oz. of pasta (I love sprouted pasta, spelt, or einkorn pasta)
- 6 carrots, diced
- 4 celery, diced
- 2 lb. chicken, diced, any kind of cut is fine
- 1 bay leaf
- 10 c. chicken broth
- 1 TBS. of my homemade italian seasoning mix
- salt & pepper to taste

DIRECTIONS:

1. Toss all ingredients EXCEPT PASTA in a slow cooker, and cook on low for 6-8 hours, or on high for 4 hours.
2. After the cooking time is done, remove bay leaf and shred chicken with a fork. Add noodles and cook an additional 20 minutes on high.

SERVES 6-8

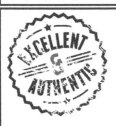

CLASSIC BEEF CHILI

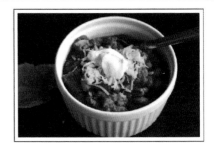

INGREDIENTS:

- 1 1/2 c. dried pinto beans
- 1 1/2 c. dried kidney beans
- 2 TBS. apple cider vinegar

- 2 TBS. tallow, lard, or coconut oil
- 1/2 large onion, diced
- 3-4 tomatoes, diced
- 1/2 pound of ground beef
- 1-6 oz. can of tomato paste
- 1-2 cubes of frozen liver
- 1 TBS. of my homemade taco seasoning
- 2 tsp. salt
- 1 TBS. of a sweetener of your choice
- 4 c. of chicken, beef or lamb broth

DIRECTIONS:

1. Place beans in a large jar or bowl and cover beans with twice as much water. Add apple cider vinegar, cover with a lid or towel and let soak for 8-12 hours on your counter top at room temperature.
2. After 8-12 hours, discard water, rinse beans well, and cook either in a pressure cooker on high pressure for 35 minutes or in a crockpot on high for 4 hours.
3. Place a big pot over medium heat on the stove top. Add tallow, onion, & ground beef. Saute for 5-10 minutes until meat is browned.
4. Add liver, tomato paste, & seasonings and mix until well combined.
5. Add beans, diced tomatoes, & broth and bring to a boil, boil for 5 minutes, then remove from heat, top with cheese & sour cream & enjoy!

SERVES 6-8

SIDE DISHES

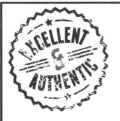

COLESLAW

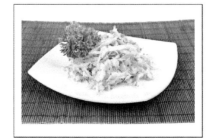

INGREDIENTS:

- 4 cups coleslaw mix
- ½ cup organic mayo
- 1 ½ tablespoon apple cider vinegar
- 1 c. diced apple
- sea salt and pepper, to taste

DIRECTIONS:

1. Mix all ingredients.
2. Refrigerate for 30 min prior to serving.

SERVES 6-8

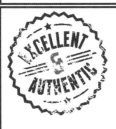

HOMEMADE GRAVY

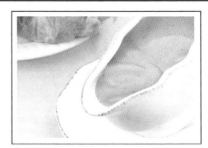

INGREDIENTS:

- 2 c. of drippings from beef, chicken, or lamb
- 1 stick butter
- 1/4 c. Organic cornstarch
- 1/2 c. cream
- 1 tsp. salt
- 1/2 tsp. pepper

DIRECTIONS:

1. In a saucepan over medium heat, melt butter.
2. Add cornstarch and whisk.
3. Add drippings, cream, salt, & pepper.
4. Once the mixture comes to a boil, remove from heat and let cool.

SERVES 6-8

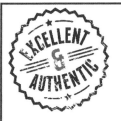

PERFECT MASHED POTATOES

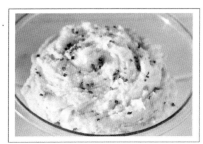

INGREDIENTS:

- 7-10 roughly peeled Organic potatoes
- 1 stick Organic butter
- 1 cup Organic cream cheese
- 1/2 cup whole Organic milk
- 1/2 tsp. onion powder
- salt & pepper to taste
- fresh chives, chopped (optional)

DIRECTIONS:

1. Start a big pot of water boiling over high heat.
2. Peel & dice potatoes.
3. Boil potatoes until a fork sticks through one easily (about 15 min.)
4. Drain all the water from the potatoes.
5. Using a mixer, blend together cooked potatoes, butter, cream cheese, 1/2 c. milk, onion powder, & salt & pepper.
6. Top with fresh chives and serve.

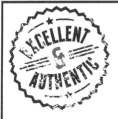

BAKED SWEET POTATOES

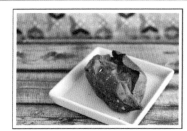

INGREDIENTS:

- 6 sweet potatoes
- 2 TBS. olive oil
- 1 tsp. sea salt

Toppings:
butter
salt n' pepper

DIRECTIONS:

1. Wash potatoes, poke a couple times with a fork, and place on a baking sheet.
2. Drizzle oilve oil & sea salt over potatoes, then bake at 350 degrees for 1 hour 15 min.
3. Remove, let cool, then add toppings and enjoy!

SERVES 6-8

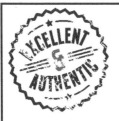

PARMESAN BROCCOLI

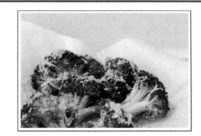

INGREDIENTS:

- 2 head of broccoli
- 3 TBS. olive oil
- 1/2 c. freshly grated parmesan
- 2 TBS. freshly grated lemon zest

DIRECTIONS:

1. Break broccoli into smaller pieces, then place on a parchment paper lined baking sheet.
2. Drizzle olive oil and sprinkle parmesan & lemon zest over broccoli.
3. Bake at 425 for 15-20 minutes or until lightly browned.

SERVES 6-8

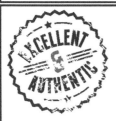

POTATO SALAD

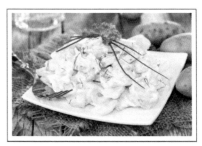

INGREDIENTS:

- 8-10 red potatoes
- 1 medium onion, diced
- 1 c. organic mayo
- 1/2 c. cream
- 1 TBS. mustard
- 1/2 tsp. garlic powder
- 1/2 tsp. onion powder
- 2 TBS. fresh dill, minced

DIRECTIONS:

1. Dice potatoes and boil in water until tender.
2. Remove potatoes from heat and drain.
3. In a small bowl, mix diced onion, mayo, cream, mustard, garlic powder, onion powder, & fresh dill.
4. Pour mixture over potatoes and fold gently.
5. Refrigerate 30 min.-1hr before serving.

SERVES 6-8

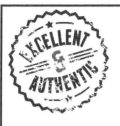

ROASTED ROOT
VEGETABLES

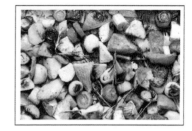

INGREDIENTS:

- 2-3 c. of any variety of root veggies
(Celery root, carrots, parsnips, sweet potatoes,
red potatoes, russet potatoes, rutabagas, turnips, etc.)
- 1/4 c. olive oil
- sea salt

DIRECTIONS:

1. Wash, peel & chop root veggies.
2. Place on a baking pan, drizzle with olive oil and sprinkle with sea salt.
3. Bake at 375 for 30-40 minutes until tender and browned.
4. Remove, let cool and enjoy!

SERVES 6-8

ROASTED & SMASHED
POTATOES

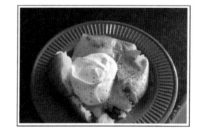

INGREDIENTS:

- 6-8 red potatoes
- 2 TBS. olive oil
- 1 tsp. sea salt

Toppings:
butter
sour cream
salt n' pepper

DIRECTIONS:

1. Wash potatoes, poke a couple times with a fork, and place in a bowl.
2. Drizzle olive oil & sea salt over potatoes, then place on a baking sheet and bake at 325 degrees for 1 hour.
3. Remove, let cool, smash down with a spatula, then add toppings and enjoy!

SERVES 6-8

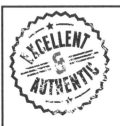

SPANISH RICE

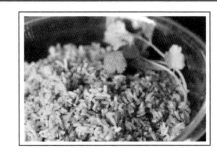

INGREDIENTS:

- 2 clove garlic, minced
- 1/2 medium onion, diced
- 3 TBS. tallow, lard, or coconut oil
- 2 c. rice (jasmine or basmati)
- 4 c. broth
- 1 TBS. tomato paste
- 1 TBS. Homemade Taco Seasoning
- 1 tsp. chili powder
- 1 TBS. honey
- 1/2 tsp. salt

DIRECTIONS:

1. Saute garlic & onion in oil for 3 minutes.
2. Add rice and toast for 5-7 minutes until light brown.
3. Add rest of ingredients, mix well and either place the entire mixture into a rice cooker or place in a saucepan, bring to a boil, then reduce & simmer on low for 18-25 minutes.

SERVES 6-8

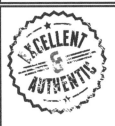

STEAMED RICE

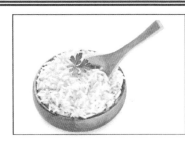

INGREDIENTS:

- 3 c. white rice (Basmati or Jasmine)
- 6 c. filtered water
- 1 TBS. butter or olive oil

DIRECTIONS:

- Rice Cooker Method: Place ingredients in rice cooker and press "cook"

- Stovetop Method: Place ingredients in a saucepan and bring to a boil then cover and simmer until done. (about 12 minutes)

SERVES 6-8

DESSERTS

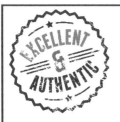

HOMEMADE PEACH
ICE CREAM

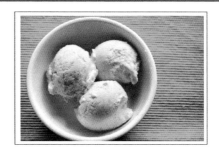

INGREDIENTS:

- 2 c. whole milk
- 1 c. heavy cream
- 2 c. peaches, preferably organic
sweetener according to your taste (maple syrup, honey, unrefined cane sugar, coconut sugar)

DIRECTIONS:

1. Place peaches (without pits) in blender and pulse until desired consistency is reached.
2. Add milk & cream and pulse until well blended.
3. Depending on how sweet your peaches are, you may not need a sweetener at all. I'll leave the amount up to you. Just taste the mixture and add according to your sweet level.
4. Place in an ice cream maker and mix until it becomes ice cream (about 20-30 minutes).

MAKES 1 QUART

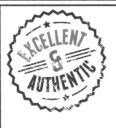

FUDGE
BROWNIES

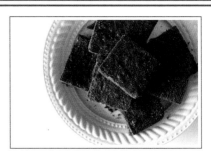

INGREDIENTS:

- 1 stick butter
- 1 cup organic cane sugar
- 2 eggs
- 1 tsp. vanilla
- 1/3 c. cocoa powder
- 1/2 c. whole wheat sprouted flour (or regular flour if you don't have any sprouted flour on hand)
- 1/4 tsp. salt
- 1/4 tsp. baking powder

DIRECTIONS:

1. Mix flour, cocoa powder, salt, baking powder in a bowl.
3. In a saucepan, melt butter just until warm, then add sugar, vanilla, eggs & whisk together. (Make sure your butter isn't too hot)
4. Add wet ingredients to dry ingredients and mix well.
5. Pour into greased 8x8 pan and bake at 350F degreed for 25 min. or until toothpick inserted comes out clean.

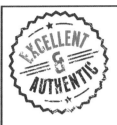

BLUEBERRY- LEMON
GELATO

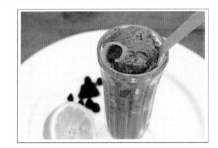

INGREDIENTS:

- 5 egg yolks
- 1/2 c. organic cane sugar or honey
- 1/4 tsp. salt
- 1/2 tsp. vanilla
- 2 1/2 c. whole milk
- 2 c. fresh or frozen blueberries
- 1 lemon

DIRECTIONS:

1. In a saucepan, combine milk & salt. While stirring occasionally, heat until it just starts to bubble.
2. Just when the milk starts to bubble, remove form heat, add vanilla, & let cool for 5 minutes.
3. Using a hand mixer or blender, blend egg yolks & sugar till creamy & well blended. Add blueberries and blend to desired consistency.
4. Slowly add milk mixture to egg/blueberry mixture.
5. Add the juice and zest of one lemon.
6. Mix till well blended, then pour into an ice cream maker and stir for aboout 20-30 minutes.

MAKES 1 QUART of GELATO

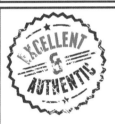

CHOCOLATE-GLAZED
SOAKED DONUTS

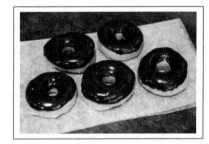

INGREDIENTS:

- 5 c. whole-wheat flour
- 2 1/4 c. warm water
- 2 TBS. acidic medium (apple cider vinegar, whey, yogurt, kefir, or lemon juice)
- 1 3/4 tsp. sea salt

- 2 heaping tsp. dry yeast
- 1 TBS. melted butter
- 1 TBS. honey
- 1/2 c. arrowroot powder, divided
- 1 c. coconut oil (for pan frying)

Chocolate Glaze
- 1/2 c. butter   - 1/4 c. whole milk
- 1 TBS. honey   - 2 tsp. real vanilla
- 3 TBS. cocoa powder - 1 1/2 c. unrefined cane sugar

DIRECTIONS:

1. Combine flour, water, 2 TBS. of acidic medium, and salt in a bowl. Mix with a spoon until well incorporated and wet.
2. Cover with a greased saran wrap and a towel tightly so it won't dry out. Leave at room temperature for 12 hours.
----
4. After 12 hours, add yeast, butter, and honey & mix well in bowl.
5. Cover again and let rise for 30 minutes.
6. Heat oil in pan over med-high heat. Sprinkle arrowroot powder generously on dough and on counter top. Roll out dough and cut into donuts.
7. Fry donuts about 45 seconds on each side until lightly browned.
8. Cool, then cover with glaze.

1. In saucepan over medium heat, melt & whisk butter, honey, cocoa powder, milk, & vanilla. Once blended, remove from heat and whisk in sugar. Coat donuts while glaze is hot.

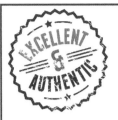

CHOCOLATE-CHIP COOKIES

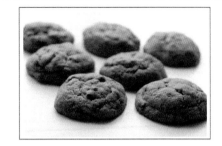

INGREDIENTS:

- 1 c. butter
- 1 c. organic cane sugar
- 1/2 c. maple syrup
- 1 tsp. real vanilla extract
- 2 eggs
- 2 1/4 c. whole wheat (sprouted is best, but regular works fine)
- 1 tsp. salt
- 1/2 tsp. baking soda
- 1/2 bag of Chocolate Chips (I like the Enjoy Life brand because they're soy free)

DIRECTIONS:

1. Preheat oven to 375F degrees. Cream butter, sugar & maple syrup.
2. Add vanilla & eggs.
3. In separate bowl, combine flour, salt, & baking soda.
4. Add dry mixture to wet mixture slowly.
5. Add chocolate chips then roll into small 2 inch balls and place on ungreased cookie sheet.
6. Bake for 8-10 minutes, and are best when cooked slightly underdone.

Makes 3 DOZEN COOKIES

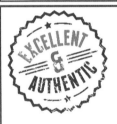

REAL FOOD HAVE YOUR CAKE CUPCAKES

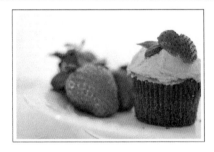

INGREDIENTS:

- 2 c. whole wheat flour (or sprouted whole wheat flour)
- 1/2 c. cocoa
- 1 1/2 TBS. baking powder
- 1/2 tsp. sea salt
- 1 1/4 c. unrefined cane sugar or coconut sugar
- 1/2 c. coconut oil or butter
- 1 2/3 c. water
- 2 eggs
- 1 TBS. vanilla

FROSTING:
- 1 pint heavy cream
- 1/4 c. powdered unrefined sugar
- 1 splash of vanilla
- 1 TBS. of beet juice for coloring (optional)

Makes 18 CUPCAKES

DIRECTIONS:

1. Mix dry ingredients well so there are no clumps.
2. Whisk wet ingredients in a separate bowl.
3. Add wet ingredients to dry and mix thoroughly.
4. Pour into lined or greased cupcake pans.
5. Bake at 325 degrees for 20-25 minutes until toothpic inserted in the center of a cupcake comes out clean.

FROSTING:
1. In a mixer, blend heavy whipping cream on high.
2. As the cream starts to thicken, slowly add sugar, vanilla, & beet juice.
3. Once the frosting has thickened, frost cooled cupcakes and devour!

FINAL THOUGHTS FROM DANELLE

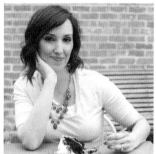 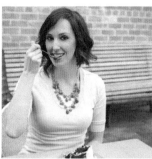 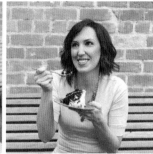 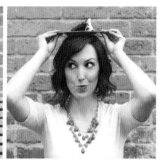

If I could give you one last bit of advice, I would say to never give up! Even if your bread falls flat on the first couple of tries, even if you can't find the best source of food, even if you fall off the wagon and eat a whole package of Oreos, just remember that it's what you do 80% of the time that matters the most! Trust me on this one! As long as you do your best to keep your home free of junk, you will succeed!

I want to thank you from the bottom of my heart for purchasing and reading my book! I have worked so hard compiling all I have learned, and I'm so grateful for the opportunity to share my knowledge with others! I hope this book helps you on your journey towards health & healing.

Please continue to follow me on my journey through real food, urban farming, & true healing on my blog at **www.weedemandreap.com**.

I have spent a lot of time and effort creating this eBook, and I ask that you do not distribute this eBook to anyone else without my permission. If you found this book useful and you would like to share with friends & family, you may share this 20% off coupon code **20SHARE.**

Again, thank you from the bottom of my heart for purchasing my book! I hope this helps you on your journey and know that I'm rooting for you!

Love,
DaNelle

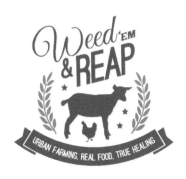

REFERENCES

Chapter 1: Real Food – how it all got messed up

Price, Weston A. Nutrition & Physical Degeneration. 2008

Ramsey, Drew. Graham, M.D. Tyler. The Happiness Diet 2012

Chapter 2: Traditional Wisdom vs. Modern Interpretation

Radford, Benjamin. Human Lifespans nearly constant for 2,000 years. Bad Science Column. 2009

Chapter 3: Modern Weight Loss Myths – Creating Confusion Since the Early 1900s.

Hargrove, Professor James L. Confusion About Calories Is Nothing New, Professor Finds. Science Daily. 2006

Quote, Mozaffarian, M.D., Dr.P.H, Dariush.

Taubes, Gary. Good Calories, Bad Calories: Fats, Carbs, and the Controversial Science of Diet and Health. 2008

Stone, Matt. Diet Recovery. 2011

Williams, Ph.D, Paul T. The National Walkers Health Study, Lawrence Berkeley National Laboratory, Life Science Division. 2013

Cook, Gray. Movement: Functional Movement Systems: Screening, Assessment, Corrective Strategies. 2011

Stone, Matt. Diet Recovery. 2011

Fallon, Sally. Enig, Mary. Nourishing Traditions: The Cookbook that Challenges Politically Correct Nutrition and the Diet Dictocrats. 1999

*Sinatra, Stephen. Bowden, **Jonny** The Great Cholesterol Myth: Why Lowering Your Cholesterol Won't Prevent Heart Disease-and the Statin-Free Plan That Will 2012*

Keys, Ancel. Anderson, Joseph T. The relationship of the diet to the development of atherosclerosis in man. 1954

Enig, Mary. Fallon, Sally. Eat Fat, Lose Fat: The Healthy Alternative to Trans Fats. 2006

Walling, Elizabeth. The Nourished Metabolism. 2013

Chapter 4: Vegan, Vegetarian, & Plant-Based Diets

Dahlin AM, Van Guelpen B, Hultdin J, Johansson I, Hallmans G, Palmqvist R. Plasma vitamin B12 concentrations and the risk of colorectal cancer: a nested case-referent study. Int J Cancer 2008;122:2057-61.

Grusack, Michael. Plant Foods as Sources of Pro-Vitamin A: Application of a Stable Isotope Approach to Determine Vitamin A Activity 2005

Schmid, Ron. Traditional Foods Are Your Best Medicine :1997

Thijssen HHW, Drittij-Reijnders MJ. Vitamin K distribution in rat tissues: dietary phylloquinone is a source of tissue menquinone-4. Br J Nutr. 1994; 72: 415-425.

Rosell MS, Lloyd-Wright Z, Appleby PN, Sanders TA, Allen NE, Key TJ. Long-chain n-3 polyunsaturated fatty acids in plasma in British meat-eating, vegetarian, and vegan men. Am J Clin Nutr.2005;82(2):327-34.

Herrmann W, Obeid R, Schorr H, Geisel J. The usefulness of holotranscobalamin in predicting vitamin B12 status in different clinical settings. Curr Drug Metab. 2005;6(1):47-53.

Daniel, Kaayla T. The Whole Soy Story: The Dark Side of America's Favorite Health Food 2005

Minger, Denise. The China Study: Fact or Fallacy?

Osteoporosis in Asia: Crossing the Frontiers, edited by E. M. C. Lau, S. C. Ho, S. Leung

Chiu, J. –F., Lan, S. –J., Yang, C.-Y., Wang, P.-W., Yaw, W. –J., and Hsieh, C. –C., Long-term vegetarian diet and bone mineral density in postmenopausal Taiwanese women, Calcified Tissue Int., 60, 245, 1997.

Hakkak, et al., "Dietary Whey Protein Protects against Azoxymethane-induced Colon Tumors in Male Rats," Cancer Epidemiology Biomarkers & Prevention, Vol. 10, 555-558, May 2001.

Spencer, Colin. The Heretic's Feast: A History of Vegetarianism. Fourth Estate Classic House, pp. 33–68, 69–84.

Chapter 5: TRUE Principles in REAL FOOD Weight Loss

Cochrane Database Syst Rev. 2003;(1):CD004022. Effects of low sodium diet versus high sodium diet on blood pressure, renin, aldosterone, catecholamines, cholesterols, and triglyceride. Jürgens G, Graudal NA.

Department of Internal Medicine and Rheumatology Q 107, Copenhagen University hospital at Herlev, Herlev Ringvej, Herlev, Copenhagen County, Denmark, 2730.

Chapter 6: Getting Started with Real Food

http://online.wsj.com/article/PR-CO-20130611-909875.html?mod=wsj_share_facebook

http://www.consumerhealth.org/articles/display.cfm?ID=20010801000231

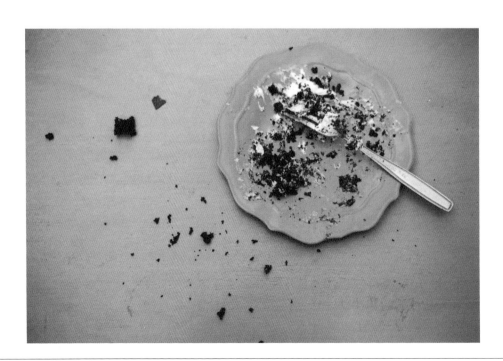

Made in the USA
Lexington, KY
05 June 2014